Exploratory Subgroup Analyses in Clinical Research,
First Edition. Gerd Rosenkranz.
© 2020 John Wiley & Sons Ltd. Published 2020 by John Wiley & Sons Ltd.
Companion website: www.wiley.com/go/rosenkranz/exploratory

Exploratory Subgroup Analyses in Clinical Research

Wiley Series on Acoustics, Noise and Vibration Series List

Formulas for Dynamics, Acoustics and Vibration Blevins
November 2015

Engineering Vibroacoustic Analysis:
Methods and Applications Hambric et al April 2016
The Effects of Sound on People Cowan May 2016

Exploratory Subgroup Analyses in Clinical Research

Gerd Rosenkranz

Statistical Consultant

WILEY

This edition first published 2020

© 2020 John Wiley & Sons Ltd

All rights reserved. No part of this publication may be reproduced, stored in a retrieval system, or transmitted, in any form or by any means, electronic, mechanical, photocopying, recording or otherwise, except as permitted by law. Advice on how to obtain permission to reuse material from this title is available at http://www.wiley.com/go/permissions.

The right of Gerd Rosenkranz to be identified as the author of this work has been asserted in accordance with law.

Registered Offices
John Wiley & Sons, Inc., 111 River Street, Hoboken, NJ 07030, USA
John Wiley & Sons Ltd, The Atrium, Southern Gate, Chichester, West Sussex, PO19 8SQ, UK

Editorial Office
9600 Garsington Road, Oxford, OX4 2DQ, UK

For details of our global editorial offices, customer services, and more information about Wiley products visit us at www.wiley.com.

Wiley also publishes its books in a variety of electronic formats and by print-on-demand. Some content that appears in standard print versions of this book may not be available in other formats.

Limit of Liability/Disclaimer of Warranty

While the publisher and authors have used their best efforts in preparing this work, they make no representations or warranties with respect to the accuracy or completeness of the contents of this work and specifically disclaim all warranties, including without limitation any implied warranties of merchantability or fitness for a particular purpose. No warranty may be created or extended by sales representatives, written sales materials or promotional statements for this work. The fact that an organization, website, or product is referred to in this work as a citation and/or potential source of further information does not mean that the publisher and authors endorse the information or services the organization, website, or product may provide or recommendations it may make. This work is sold with the understanding that the publisher is not engaged in rendering professional services. The advice and strategies contained herein may not be suitable for your situation. You should consult with a specialist where appropriate. Further, readers should be aware that websites listed in this work may have changed or disappeared between when this work was written and when it is read. Neither the publisher nor authors shall be liable for any loss of profit or any other commercial damages, including but not limited to special, incidental, consequential, or other damages.

Library of Congress Cataloging-in-Publication Data

Names: Rosenkranz, Gerd, 1955- author.
Title: Exploratory subgroup analyses in clinical research / Gerd
   Rosenkranz.
Other titles: Statistics in practice.
Description: Hoboken, NJ : Wiley, 2020. | Series: Wiley series in
   statistics in practice | Includes bibliographical references and index.
Identifiers: LCCN 2019051500 (print) | LCCN 2019051501 (ebook) | ISBN
   9781119536970 (hardback) | ISBN 9781119536956 (adobe pdf) | ISBN
   9781119537007 (epub)
Subjects: MESH: Cluster Analysis | Clinical Trials as Topic | Models,
   Statistical | Precision Medicine
Classification: LCC R853.C55 (print) | LCC R853.C55 (ebook) | NLM WA 950
   | DDC 610.72/4--dc23
LC record available at https://lccn.loc.gov/2019051500
LC ebook record available at https://lccn.loc.gov/2019051501

ISBN: 9781119536970

Cover Design: Wiley
Cover Image: Gerd Rosenkranz Figure 7.5

Set in 13/15.5pt, PhotinaMTStd by SPi Global, Chennai, India.

10 9 8 7 6 5 4 3 2 1

*To my parents,
Ruth and Karl*

Contents

Preface xi
Acknowledgments xiii
Acronyms xv
About the Companion Website xix
Introduction xxi

1 Some History of Subgroup Analysis 1

   1.1 Introduction 1
   1.2 Questionable Subgroup Analyses 5
       1.2.1 Star Signs May Matter 5
       1.2.2 Unjustified Under-treatment 7
       1.2.3 Misinterpretation of Center Effects 8
       1.2.4 The End of a Career 10
   1.3 Encouraging Subgroup Analyses 12
       1.3.1 Higher Efficacy 12
       1.3.2 Harm Prevention 13
       1.3.3 Avoiding Unnecessary Treatment 16
   1.4 Subgroups and Drug Approvals 18
       1.4.1 A Convincing Subgroup 18
       1.4.2 Inconsistencies Across Regions 19
       1.4.3 Detecting Non-responders 22
       1.4.4 In Search for Benefit 26
   1.5 Concluding Remarks 29

2 Objectives and Current Practice of Subgroup Analyses — 31

- 2.1 Introduction — 31
- 2.2 Objectives of Subgroup Analyses — 32
- 2.3 Definitions Around Subgroups — 34
- 2.4 Confounding — 37
- 2.5 Two Types of Subgroup Analyses — 39
- 2.6 Reporting of Subgroups — 43
- 2.7 Concluding Remarks — 45

3 Pitfalls of Subgroup Analyses — 47

- 3.1 Introduction — 47
- 3.2 Extreme Effect Estimates — 48
- 3.3 Selection Bias — 51
- 3.4 Reversal of Effects — 53
- 3.5 Regression to the Mean — 57
- 3.6 Simpson's Paradox — 60
- 3.7 Post-hoc Analyses — 63
- 3.8 Concluding Remarks — 65

4 Subgroup Analysis and Modeling — 67

- 4.1 Introduction — 67
- 4.2 Modeling and Prediction — 69
- 4.3 Subgroups and Hierarchical Models — 72
  - 4.3.1 Stein's Discovery — 72
  - 4.3.2 The Normal–Normal Hierarchical Model — 73
- 4.4 Subgroups and Regression Models — 76
  - 4.4.1 Subgroups Defined in Terms of Variables — 76
  - 4.4.2 The Predicted Individual Treatment Effect — 79
  - 4.4.3 Comparison of the Two Options — 83
- 4.5 Variable Selection in Regression — 85
  - 4.5.1 Classical Variable Selection — 86

	4.5.2	Regularized Estimators	87
	4.5.3	Variable Selection and Confounding	88
4.6	Concluding Remarks		89

5 Hierarchical Models in Subgroup Analysis — 91

5.1	Introduction		91
5.2	A General Hierarchical Model		94
	5.2.1	Robbins' Theorem and Tweedie's Formula	94
	5.2.2	Mixture Priors	97
	5.2.3	The False Discovery Rate	100
5.3	Parameter Estimation		101
	5.3.1	Posterior Means and Variances	101
	5.3.2	Estimation Bias	104
	5.3.3	Selection Bias	106
5.4	Case Studies		111
	5.4.1	The Toxoplasmosis Dataset	111
	5.4.2	The BCG Dataset	113
	5.4.3	The Prostate Cancer Dataset	119
5.5	Concluding Remarks		124

6 Selection Bias in Regression — 129

6.1	Introduction	129
6.2	Correction for Selection Bias	131
6.3	Variance Estimation	136
6.4	A Case Study	139
6.5	Concluding Remarks	144

7 The Predicted Individual Treatment Effect — 147

7.1	Introduction	148
7.2	Definition of the PITE	149

x   *Contents*

7.3	Confidence Intervals of the PITE		150
	7.3.1	MLE for the Full Model	151
	7.3.2	MLE Under a Reduced Model	151
	7.3.3	Scheffé Confidence Bounds	152
	7.3.4	LASSO with Post-selection Intervals	152
	7.3.5	Randomized LASSO	154
	7.3.6	Simulation Study	154
	7.3.7	Extension to Other Endpoints	157
7.4	Case Studies		159
	7.4.1	An Alzheimer Dataset	160
	7.4.2	The Prostate Cancer Study Again	161
	7.4.3	Renal Safety of Contrast Media	165
7.5	Concluding Remarks		173

8   Prediction models   175

8.1	Introduction	176
8.2	Prediction Error	177
8.3	Model Selection or Averaging	180
8.4	Prediction Error of the PITE	182
8.5	A Case Study	187
8.6	Concluding Remarks	190

9   Outlook   193

Bibliography   **197**

Index   **217**

Preface

A few years ago I started a book by first writing a fairly extensive preface. I never finished that book and resolved that in the future I would write first the book and then the preface.

Leo Breiman (1928–2005)
—Preface to "Probability" (Breiman, 1968)

When I eventually agreed to write a book on subgroup analyses I remembered the first paragraph of the preface that the late (and great) probabilist and statistician Leo Breiman added to his book "Probability," a classic textbook during my study days. I interpreted Leo's words as a warning to all potential authors not to start from the wrong end. Hence I postponed writing this part of the book if not to the very end but to the point when progress looked encouraging.

This book is about a topic of intense research driven on one hand by the promises of precision medicine and on the other by the intention of regulating agencies to obtain information about the consistency of findings from clinical trials in drug applications. It can therefore be at best a snapshot of the state of the art at a given point in time from the author's perspective of the topic.

To whom may the book concern? First, its main parts require a solid knowledge of statistical concepts like random variables, bias, variance, confidence intervals, and statistical tests, but also a background in statistical modeling, re-sampling, and model selection. Re-sampling is well presented in "An Introduction to the Bootstrap" (Efron and Tibshirani, 1993) while "Statistical Learning with Sparsity" (Hastie et al., 2015) covers the modern aspects of modeling and model selection.

On the practical side, knowledge about concepts of clinical trials and drug development like efficacy and safety, and randomization and blinding are helpful. "Statistical Issues in Drug Development" (Senn, 2007) covers many of these topics.

Notwithstanding what is said above, parts of the book should be readable by a non-statistical audience, mainly the chapters on history and to a lesser extent on pitfalls. Chapters digging a bit deeper into methodology (those coming with a heavier load of equations) should be primarily appreciated by statisticians. With this in mind, clinicians and statisticians from the area of clinical development and regulation should benefit most, although the topic of subgroup analysis has a much wider scope.

Lörrach, Germany GERD K. ROSENKRANZ
April 2019

Acknowledgments

Part of the work presented here was developed while I was employed with Novartis Pharma AG in Basel, Switzerland, in cooperation with an EFSPI Working Group on subgroup analyses led by Aaron Dane (DaneStat) and later by David Svensson (AstraZeneca). I thank both Aaron and David, as well as Amy Spencer (University of Sheffield) and Ilya Lipkovich (IQVIA, now Lilly) from this group for their cooperation. The results of this group are presented in Dane et al. (2019). I would like to thank specifically Björn Bornkamp (Novartis) for many discussions on subgroup selection and modeling.

The topic was developed further during a two-year visiting professorship at the Center of Medical Statistics, Informatics and Intelligent Systems at the Medical University of Vienna, for which I am really grateful to Martin Posch, the center director, and to Franz König. The hospitality at the Institute and the cooperation with colleagues, in particular with our then PhD student Nicolas

Ballarini, added new motivation to keep working on the topic with new drive and direction. Having had the opportunity to work and live in the city of Vienna was really a privilege. Sincere thanks also to Thomas Jaki (University of Lancaster) for providing funding from the UK Medical Research Council, Project No. MR/M005755/1 during this time.

My involvement in the subgroup topic got on the radar screen of Alison Oliver from John Wiley after a half day seminar I presented at ISCB 2016 in Birmingham, UK. Without her indefatigable reminders to make up my mind and agree on a book project this would have hardly happened.

Last but not least I would like to thank my parents who gave me (and my brother) the opportunity and the support to complete an education of our choice. I also want to thank my wife for accepting the seemingly endless hours I withdrew to work at the laptop in my home office.

GERD K. ROSENKRANZ

Acronyms

ASA	Acetylsalicylic acid
AIC	Akaike information criterion
ATE	Average treatment effect
BHAT	Beta-Blocker Heart Attack Trial
BIC	Bayesian information criterion
CAPRIE	Clopidogrel versus aspirin in patients at risk of Ischemic events
cdf	Cumulative distribution function
CONSORT	Consolidated Standards of Reporting Trials
DILI	Drug induced liver injury
EB	Empirical Bayes
EGFR	Epidermal growth factor receptor
EMA	European Medicines Agency
FDA	Food and Drug Administration
Fdr	False discovery rate
GISSI	Gruppo Italiano per lo Studio della Streptochinasi nell'Infarcto Miocardico
GLIM	Generalized linear model
HAMD	Hamilton depression rating scale

HER2	Human epidermal growth factor receptor 2
IPF	Idiopathic pulmonary fibrosis
IQWiQ	Institute for Quality and Efficiency in Healthcare
ITT	Intention to treat
ISIS	International Study of Infarct Survival
KM	Kaplan–Meier
KRAS	Kirsten Rat Sarcoma viral oncogene analog
Lasso	Least absolute shrinkage and selection operator
MARS	Montgomery–Asberg depression rating scale
ME	Model error
MLE	Maximum likelihood estimator
MERIT-HF	Metoprolol controlled release randomized intervention trial in heart failure
MHLW	Ministry of Health, Labor and Welfare
NICE	National Institute of Health and Clinical Excellence
pdf	Probability density function
PE	Prediction error
PEP	Prediction error of the PITE
PITE	Predicted individual treatment effect
PLATO	Platelet Inhibition and Clinical Outcomes Trial
PMDA	Pharmaceuticals and Medical Devices Agency

RSE	Residual squared error
r.v.	Random variable(s)
SE	Standard error
TARGET	Therapeutic Arthritis Research and Gastrointestinal Event Trial
TAYLORx	Trial Assigning Individualized Options for Treatment
TMS	Transcranial magnetic stimulation

About the Companion Website

This book is accompanied by a companion website:

www.wiley.com/go/rosenkranz/exploratory

The website includes:
Datasets and Programs.

Scan this QR code to visit the companion website.

Introduction

The promise of precision medicine is to identify subgroups of patients that respond better to treatment than the patient population as a whole. This idea is particularly relevant for new anticancer agents that target specific molecular pathways (Karapetis et al., 2008). Since treatments targeting specific pathways are becoming more prominent in other indications as well, the quest for predictive markers increases (Slager et al., 2012; Buck and Hemmer, 2014).

The topic is also of interest in a broader regulatory context. In a recent guideline, the European Medicines Agency (EMA, 2019) states that investigation into the effects of treatment in well-defined subsets of the trial population is an integral part of clinical trial planning, analysis, and inference that follows the inspection of the primary outcome of the trial. The intention is to investigate consistency or heterogeneity of the treatment effect across subgroups defined in terms of background characteristics.

As early as 1988 the Food and Drug Administration (FDA) of the United States issued regulations on the content and format of new drug applications (FDA, 1988) that require the presentation of effectiveness and safety data by gender, age, and racial subgroups, and the identification of dosage modifications for specific subgroups. In 2014, the FDA published an action plan to enhance the collection and availability of demographic subgroup data (FDA, 2014).

Subgroup analysis poses issues (Assmann et al., 2000; Senn, 2001; Wang et al., 2007) and can be controversial, in particular in regard to findings after the fact; see debates in Horwitz et al. (1996,1997), Senn and Harrell (1997), Bender et al. (2010), and Hasford et al. (2010,2011). Nevertheless there are good arguments to investigate a potential heterogeneity of treatment effect, for example in relation to pathophysiology (Rothwell, 2005).

The focus of the book is a situation where some, but not too many subgroups like gender, age, region, disease severity, ethnic origin, metabolism etc., have been identified at the trial outset to be examined in an exploratory way when the data are available. Identifying subgroups encompasses searching for a feature that is sticking out, for example an extraordinary treatment or side effect. This entails a two-fold risk of wrongly selecting subgroups and of overestimating the effect size in the selected subgroup(s). (Adjustment for multiplicity can cope with the risk of too many false positive results, but not automatically with selection bias.) The statistical problem has become known as "selective inference", the assessment of relevance and effect sizes from a dataset after mining the same data to find associations (Taylor and Tibshirani, 2015).

It has been pointed out by several authors (Assmann et al., 2000; Rothwell, 2005) that the correct criterion to identify subgroups with higher treatment effects is not the significance of the treatment effect in one subgroup or the other, but whether the effect differs between the subgroups defined by a factor, i.e. a treatment by factor or treatment by subgroup interaction. However, a test for this interaction suffers from the fact that it may come out significant for minor interactions when the sample size is large, while it may tend to miss large interactions when the sample size is small. Hence other methods may be required to address subgroup identification.

The book is organized as follows. First we take a guided tour through the history of subgroup analyses and introduce subgroup analyses that actually happened and are each remarkable for a special reason. This part of the book should be readable (and understandable) by a broad audience beyond statisticians.

Next we summarize the objectives of subgroup analyses and present definitions around subgroups. Some of the most prominent pitfalls of subgroup analyses are discussed in Chapter 3 followed by an introduction of different methods to analyze data from subgroups: hierarchical models to reduce variability of estimators (Chapter 5), application of the bootstrap to reduce bias in effect estimators after subgroup selection (Chapter 6), methods to obtain estimates of expected individual treatment effects (Chapter 7) and prediction errors in prediction models (Chapter 8). The presentation of methods for subgroup analyses includes illustrative case studies.

ard # 1

Some History of Subgroup Analysis

> *The essence of tragedy has been described as the destructive collision of two sets of protagonists, both of whom are correct. The statisticians are right in denouncing subgroups that are formed post hoc from exercises in pure data dredging. The clinicians are also right, however, in insisting that a subgroup is respectable and worthwhile when established a priori from pathophysiological principles. (Feinstein, 1998)*

Alvan R Feinstein (1925–2001)

The Problem of Cogent Subgroups: A Clinicostatistical Tragedy.

1.1 INTRODUCTION

The history of subgroup analysis is characterized by a strong difference in opinions about its value.

2　Some History of Subgroup Analysis

One group of scientists has a skeptical attitude towards the topic warning of the risks of subgroup analysis and other attempts to target treatments. For example, Yusuf et al. (1984) stated that "... it would be unfortunate if desire for the perfect (i.e. knowledge of exactly who will benefit from treatment) were to become the enemy of the possible (i.e. knowledge of the direction and approximate size of the effects of treatment of wide categories of patients)." Many clinicians are afraid of applying the overall results of large trials to individual patients without consideration of determinants of individual responses (Rothwell, 2005) while most prominently statisticians have raised concerns (Assmann et al., 2000, Sleight, 2000, Lagakos, 2006, Guillemin, 2007, Lonergan et al., 2017) and requested that:

- Investigators should be cautious when undertaking subgroup analyses.
- Subgroup findings should be exploratory, and only exceptionally should they affect the conclusions from trials.
- Editors and reviewers of journals need to correct any inappropriate, over-enthusiastic uses of subgroup analyses.

The statement "subgroups kill people" was attributed – rightly or wrongly – to statistician Sir Richard Peto in van Gijn and Algra (1994). In fact, Peto commented on subgroup analyses undertaken on the GISSI[1] study (GISSI Study Group, 1986): "The GISSI study ... is one of the most important randomized trials ever conducted and when it was published provided the best evidence then available that thrombolytic therapy reduced mortality. But the ability of the GISSI report to save lives could be substantially compromised by misinterpretation by clinicians of some of the data-dependent subset analyses that it contained." (Peto, 1990)

A second camp of scientists and pharmaceutical executives is more attracted by the opportunities than by the risks of subgroup analysis driven by the vision of "personalized" medicine. In 1977, Sir Richard Sykes, at the time chief executive officer of Glaxo-Wellcome, later chairman of GlaxoSmith-Kline and rector of Imperial College London, wrote:

"It will soon be possible for patients in clinical trials to undergo genetic tests to identify those individuals who will respond favorably to the drug candidate, based on their genotype, and therefore the underlying mechanism of their disease. This will translate into smaller, more effective clinical trials with corresponding cost savings and ultimately better treatment in general practice. In addition, clinical trials will be capable of screening for genes involved in the absorption, metabolism and clearance of drugs and the genes that are

---

[1] GISSI = Gruppo Italiano per lo Studio della Streptochinasi nell'Infarcto Miocardico

likely to predispose a patient to drug-induced side-effects. In this way, individual patients will be targeted with specific treatment and personalized dosing regimens to maximize efficacy and minimize pharmacokinetic problems and other side-effects." (Sykes, 1977), quoted from Senn (2001). It took another 20+ years until the first targeted medicine in oncology, trastuzumab for HER2 positive breast cancer, was approved by the US Food and Drug Administration (FDA) in 1998.

More and more drugs were approved for targeted patient populations during the following years. A selective list is displayed in Table 1.1. In 2013, the FDA issued a report "Paving the way to personalized medicine" (FDA, 2013) describing how the agency was planning to support the development of new drugs with companion

Table 1.1 Approved targeted therapies

Indication	Marker	Compound
Breast cancer	HER2+	trastuzumab
		pertuzumab
	HER2-/ER+	everolimus
Colorectal cancer	KRAS	cetuximab
		panatumumab
Cystic fibrosis	G551D	ivacaftor
Melanoma	BRAF V600E	vemurafenib
		dabrafenib
	BRAF V600E or V600K	trametinib
NSCLC	ALK	crizotinib

1.2 QUESTIONABLE SUBGROUP ANALYSES

1.2.1 Star Signs May Matter

A trial that Peto mentioned in his critique on the GISSI study to justify his concerns on subgroup analyses was ISIS–2[2] (ISIS–2 Collaborative Group, 1988). This study enrolled 17 187 patients in 417 hospitals up to 24 h after the onset of suspected myocardial infarction. Patients were randomized to (i) a one hour iv infusion of streptokinase; (ii) one month of 160 mg/day aspirin; (iii) both active treatments; or (iv) neither. In the end, streptokinase reduced five week vascular mortality by $25 \pm 4\%$ as compared to placebo ($2p < 0.00001$). Aspirin reduced five week vascular mortality by $23 \pm 4\%$ as compared to placebo ($2p < 0.00001$). The combination of both aspirin and streptokinase reduced five week vascular mortality by $45 \pm 5\%$ as compared to placebo ($2p < 0.00001$).

The study authors concluded on subgroup analyses: "Even in a trial as large as ISIS–2, reliable identification of subgroups of patients among whom treatment is particularly advantageous (or among whom it is ineffective) is unlikely to be

---

[2]ISIS = International Study of Infarct Survival

possible. When in a trial with a clearly positive overall result many subgroup analyses are considered, false negative results in some particular subgroups must be expected." They underlined their opinion with "the most entertaining example of an inappropriate subgroup analysis" (Horton, 2000): "For example, subdivision of the patients in ISIS–2 with respect to their astrological birth signs appears to indicate that for patients born under Gemini or Libra there was a slightly adverse effect of aspirin on mortality (9% ± 13% odds increase; NS), while for patients born under all other astrological signs there was a strikingly beneficial effect (28% ± 5%) odds reduction; $2p < 0.00001$)." The results for the aspirin–placebo comparison are shown in Table 1.2

The reason for this odd item appearing in the paper originated in negotiations between authors and editors. The Lancet was keen to include clinically relevant subgroup findings. The authors agreed under the proviso that the journal allowed

Table 1.2 Vascular deaths in the ISIS–2 study

Star sign	Aspirin			Placebo			Odds ratio
	N	deaths	(%)	N	deaths	(%)	
Gemini/ Libra	1357	150	11.1	1442	147	10.2	1.09
Other	7228	654	9.0	7157	868	12.1	0.72

Source: ISIS–2 Collaborative Group (1988)

the star sign groups to appear first to underline for readers the reliance they might put (or not) on the validity of these analyses (Horton, 2000).

1.2.2 Unjustified Under-treatment

The artificial subgroup analysis just described has at least one real world counterpart that caused serious under-treatment of a subgroup of patients for at least a decade because of a subgroup analysis: a Canadian Cooperative Study Group trial came to the conclusion that aspirin was effective in preventing stroke and death in men but not in women. The gender by treatment interaction turned out to be significant ($p = 0.003$) and aspirin was effective in preventing stroke and death in men (RR= 0.52, $p < 0.005$) but not in women (1.42, $p = 0.35$) (The Canadian Cooperative Study Group, 1978).

As part of a major meta-analysis of studies of high risk subjects in which individual patient data were obtained it was concluded that antiplatelet therapy for high risk patients appeared to reduce the odds of vascular events by a roughly similar proportion regardless of age or gender of the subjects (Antiplatelet Trialists' Collaboration, 1994). Thus the notion that women might not benefit from antiplatelet therapy (which arose from data dependent subgroup analyses of a few trials) is contradicted by much more reliable, prospectively planned overview analyses.

1.2.3 Misinterpretation of Center Effects

Most randomized controlled clinical trials are conducted in multiple centers since a single center is unable to provide all of the necessary patients for a definitive study, for example, when the condition under study is rare or the anticipated treatment effect is small. A controversy that has emerged concerning the analysis of multi-center trials is the interpretation of divergent center results. In a post hoc analysis of the Beta-Blocker Heart Attack Trial (BHAT), Horwitz et al. (1996) illustrated the occurrence of substantial variation in results among the participating centers.

BHAT enrolled 3837 subjects in 31 clinical centers in the United States and Canada. Eligible subjects included men and women between the ages of 30 and 39 years who had been hospitalized with an acute myocardial infarction. Patients were randomized to receive propanolol or a matching placebo after their condition had stabilized. The minimum length of follow-up was 12 months and the average time on trial was 25 months. Overall, 1916 subjects were randomized to propanolol and 1921 to placebo. At 25 months the estimated mortality rates were 7.2% for propanolol and 9.8% for placebo, for a relative risk of 0.73 and a 95% confidence interval (CI)= (0.59, 0.90).

In the course of a post hoc investigation, Horwitz et al. (1996) divided the centers into two groups: 21 dominant centers in which mortality rates were higher for patients on placebo and 10 divergent centers in which higher mortality rates occurred for patients on propanolol. The relative risk in the dominant centers favoring propanolol was 0.5, 95% CI= (0.38, 0.67). In the divergent centers, they obtained a relative risk of 1.33 and a 95% CI= (0.95, 1.88). These numbers are summarized in Table 1.3.

The test for qualitative interactions by Gail and Simon (1985) was significant on the 5% level supporting the view of the authors that propanolol is potentially helpful for patients in the dominant centers and potentially harmful for the diverging centers.

This view was criticized in a dissent by Senn and Harrell (1997) who were not at all surprised that Horwitz et al. (1996) found a significant difference between the two groups of centers. In fact they argued that "a very similar analysis applied to *any multicenter trial whatsoever* will always be significant at the 5% level provided only that the

Table 1.3 Results from BHAT by center subgroups and overall

Subgroup	Number of subjects	Relative risk (95% CI)
21 dominant centers	2480	0.50 (0.38, 0.67)
10 divergent centers	1357	1.33 (0.95, 1.88)
All centers	3837	0.73 (0.59, 0.90)

Source: Horwitz et al. (1996)

number of centers is at least equal to 8." The analysis they proposed was to rank the centers according to the treatment effect, divide them into two groups above and below the median and carry out a rank test on the groups so defined.

They argued further that given the overall mortality rates of 0.072 and 0.098 for the treatment and control group, no heterogeneity between centers and an average center size of 62, one obtains a probability of an effect reversal favoring control of 0.25 per center. The expected number of effect reversal for a trial of 31 centers of equal size would then amount to $0.25 \times 31 = 7.7$ and the probability of 10 or more effect reversals would be 0.22. They also complain about the improper use of the Gail–Simon test (Gail and Simon, 1985), which requires subsets to be specified in advance and not based on observed event rate differences.

In a rejoinder, Horwitz et al. (1997) re-iterated that the results of clinical trials providing average effects on intention to treat (ITT) patient populations that ignore post randomization interventions do not support the needs of treating physicians to prescribe the best treatment for an individual patient.

1.2.4 The End of a Career

A study that had a material impact on the players involved was the Actimmune trial in idiopathic pulmonary fibrosis (IPF) (Raghu et al., 2004). The study enrolled 330 IPF patients who were randomized between placebo and Actimmune (Interferon gamma-1b). At the study conclusion, no significant difference in the primary endpoint (progression free survival) nor in any of nine secondary endpoints could be found. However, the mortality rate was 40% lower under the test treatment compared to placebo ($p = 0.084$). In addition, in a post hoc subgroup of 254 patients with mild to moderate disease, mortality was reduced by 70% ($p = 0.004$).

The company issued a press release[3] entitled "InterMune announces Phase III Data Demonstrating Survival Benefit of Actimmune in IPF: Reduces Mortality by 70% in Patients With Mild to Moderate Disease" with the following conclusions:

- "Preliminary data ... demonstrate a significant survival benefit in patients with mild to moderate disease randomly assigned to Actimmune versus the control treatment ($p = 0.004$)."

- "There was also approximately a 10% relative reduction in the rate of progression-free survival associated with Actimmune versus placebo, the trial's primary endpoint, but this was not a statistically significant difference."

InterMune then promoted the drug off-label in IPF, while the FDA never approved it in this indication. In 2003, the company initiated the INSPIRE trial, a study of Actimmune in patients

[3] http://www.sec.gov/Archives/edgar/data/1087432/ 000091205702033878/a2088367zex-99_1.htm

with mild to moderate IPF to confirm the results of the post hoc subgroup analysis. Unfortunately, the study was terminated in 2007 after an interim analysis showed no survival benefit. InterMune sold the drug in 2012.

The CEO of InterMune was prosecuted by the US Department of Justice for " ... fraudulently promoting the drug Actimmune", by issuing " ... false and misleading information about the drugs effectiveness in treating idiopathic pulmonary fibrosis." In 2009 the CEO was found guilty of wire fraud by a jury. The conviction was affirmed by the Ninth Circuit of the United States Court of Appeals in March 2013 and a petition for writ of certiorari was denied by the US Supreme Court in December 2013.

1.3 ENCOURAGING SUBGROUP ANALYSES

1.3.1 Higher Efficacy

The growth factor receptor HER2 is over-expressed in 25 to 30% of breast cancers, increasing the aggressiveness of the tumor. To evaluate the efficacy and safety of trastuzumab, a recombinant monoclonal antibody against HER2, in women with metastatic breast cancer over-expressing HER2, 469 patients were enrolled in a prospective clinical study, 234 of whom were randomized to receive standard chemotherapy and 235 to receive standard chemotherapy plus trastuzumab. Patients who had not previously received adjuvant therapy with an anthracycline were treated with doxorubicin or epirubicine in combination with cyclophosphamide with (143 women) or without (138 women) trastuzumab. Patients who had previously been treated with anthracyclines were treated with paclitaxel alone (96 woman) or paclitaxel plus trastuzumab (92 woman). The addition of trastuzumab was associated with a longer time to disease progression, a higher rate of objective response and a higher one year survival rate (Slamon et al., 2001). The results for time to progression (primary endpoint) and mortality are summarized in Table 1.4.

The interesting feature of this study is that it included only patients with HER2 positive cancer, i.e. exclusively the predefined subgroup, without a direct comparison in HER2 negative tumors. The evidence that trastuzumab would be primarily efficacious in HER2 positive disease was obtained from earlier studies.

1.3.2 Harm Prevention

Idiosyncratic drug-induced liver injury (DILI) is a major safety concern and has been a common cause for the marketing withdrawal of a range of drugs. Due to the unpredictable and rare nature of these events it is often not until the post-marketing phase that a drug's propensity for DILI is revealed.

Table 1.4 Results on time to progression and survival from the trastuzumab study in HER2 positive breast cancer

End point	C+T	C	A+T	A	P+T	P
Median time to disease progression (months)	7.4	4.6	7.8	6.1	6.9	3.0
—Relative risk of progression (95% CI)	0.51 (0.41–0.63)		0.62 (0.47–0.81)		0.38 (0.27–0.53)	
—p-value	<0.001		<0.001		<0.001	
Median survival time (months)	25.1	20.3	26.8	21.4	22.1	18.4
—Relative risk of death (95% CI)	0.80 (0.64–1.00)		0.82 (0.61–1.09)		0.80 (0.56–1.11)	
—p-value	0.046		0.16		0.17	

C+T = chemotherapy plus trastuzumab, C = chemotherapy alone, A+T = anthracycline plus trastuzumab, A = anthracycline alone, P+T = paclitaxel plus trastuzumab, P = paclitaxel alone. Time to progression and survival were analyzed nine months and 31 months after enrollment of the last patient, respectively. Source: Slamon et al. (2001)

The discovery of genetic markers able to identify individuals at risk could make otherwise safe and efficacious drugs available for use.

Concerns over hepatoxicity have contributed to the withdrawal or non-approval of the selective COX-2 inhibitor lumiracoxib, which proved to be efficacious in osteoarthritis and acute pain (Bannwarth and Berenbaum, 2007). To identify genetic markers able to select individuals at risk for developing drug induced liver injury a case-control genome-wide association study was conducted in 41 lumiracoxib treated patients with liver enzyme elevations above five times the upper limit of normal (ULN) and 176 patients without liver injury (Singer et al., 2010) using DNA samples collected from the TARGET[4] study (Farkouh et al., 2004). Endpoints were time to liver enzyme elevations above five times ULN. Fine mapping identified a strong association with a common HLA haplotype. HLA-DQA1*0102 had the best results in terms of negative predictive value (99%) and sensitivity (73.6%).

To further examine the performance characteristics of the marker, all remaining 4518 lumiracoxib treated patients from the TARGET study with DNA available who had given informed consent were genotyped for the presence or absence of HLA-DQA1*0102. Kaplan–Meier (KM) estimates of the cumulative incidence

---

[4]TARGET = Therapeutic Arthritis Research and Gastrointestinal Event Trial

of liver enzyme elevations were obtained for HLA-DQA1*0102 carriers and non-carriers and compared to estimates for all patients treated with lumiracoxib, ibuprofen or naproxen. As it turns out, the KM curve for lumiracoxib treated subjects who are DQA*0102 carriers is increasing much faster over time than the KMs for patients treated with the comparator drugs. The risk of non-carriers under lumiracoxib is similar to the risk in the overall population under the comparator treatments (Figure 2 in Singer et al. (2010)). The paper concludes: "The results presented here provide strong evidence that the HLA-DQA1*0102 allele would have clinical utility as a screening marker to exclude carriers from lumiracoxib treatment." In any case, the study moved the field of personalized medicine into the safety area with one of the first DILI safety markers.

1.3.3 Avoiding Unnecessary Treatment

Hormone-receptor-positive, axillary node-negative disease accounts for approximately half of all cases of breast cancer in the United States. Adjuvant chemotherapy reduces the risk of recurrence with effects greater in younger women. These findings let a National Institute of Health (NIH) panel recommend adjuvant chemotherapy for most patients, leading to a declining breast cancer mortality. However, the majority of patients may receive chemotherapy unnecessarily.

A recurrence score ranging from 0 to 100 based on the 21-gene breast cancer assay (OncotypeDX) predicts chemotherapy benefit if it is high and a low risk of recurrence without chemotherapy if it is low (Sparano and Paik, 2008, Sparano et al., 2015). However, there was uncertainty about benefit of chemotherapy for most patients who have a midrange score. To close this knowledge gap, the National Cancer Institute (NCI) sponsored the Trial Assigning Individualized Options for Treatment (TAILORx) (Sparano et al., 2018).

TAILORx was a prospective trial involving 10273 women with hormone-receptor-positive, human epidermal growth factor receptor 2 (HER2)-negative, axillary node-negative breast cancer. Of the 9719 eligible patients, 6711 had a midrange recurrence score of 11 to 25. These subjects were randomly assigned to either chemoendocrine therapy or endocrine therapy alone. The trial was designed to show non-inferiority of endocrine therapy alone for invasive disease-free survival, defined as freedom from invasive disease recurrence, second primary cancer or death. A five year rate of invasive disease-free survival rate of 90% with chemoendocrine therapy and of 87% or less with endocrine therapy alone, which corresponds to a hazard ration of 1.322, was specified as unacceptable.

After conclusion of the trial, the hazard ratio for invasive disease-free survival of endocrine relative to chemoendocrine therapy was 1.08 with a 95% confidence interval of (0.94, 1.24).

Non-inferiority could also be concluded in other endpoints. A significant interaction between age and chemotherapy treatment was found that confirmed previous findings. However, it is unclear whether the string of covariates underlying the exploratory analyses were pre-specified. The study confirmed the generally good results for scores below 10 on endocrine therapy alone and the slightly worse results under chemoendocrine treatment for scores of 26 and above.

1.4 SUBGROUPS AND DRUG APPROVALS

1.4.1 A Convincing Subgroup

In 2008, the Food and Drug Administration (FDA) cleared the first transcranial magnetic stimulation (TMS) device to treat depression in patients who failed on one antidepressant. In an editorial (Hines et al., 2009), the authors raised concerns that the decision was based on a post hoc subgroup analysis of a published negative randomized controlled trial (O'Reardon et al., 2007), re-analyzed by Lisanby et al. (2009).

In the double-blind study, 301 patients with major depression who had not benefited from prior treatment were randomized; 155 to active and 146 to sham TMS. The primary outcome was a change from baseline to week 4 on the

Montgomery–Asberg depression rating scale (MADRS).

The difference between treatment groups was 1.7 points on the 60 points MARDS at four weeks with a *p*-value of 0.057, "both statistically and clinically non-significant." (Hines et al., 2009). The finding became significant ($p = 0.038$) after the post hoc exclusion of six patients with baseline MADRS below 20. In the result section of the publication, the authors claimed that "active TMS was significantly superior to sham TMS on the MADRS (with a post hoc correction for inequality in symptom severity between groups at baseline)."

When presented with these data, the FDA Advisory Committee concluded that TMS' "clinical effect was perhaps marginal, borderline, questionable, and perhaps a reasonable person could ask whether there was an effect at all" and rejected the device. FDA overruled its committee and granted approval. In the agency's favor it may be argued that the original result was close to significance and that subjects with low MARDS at baseline do not have a good chance to improve. This may impact the results if these subjects are not evenly distributed amongst treatment groups. However, an analysis of covariance may have been an alternative option.

1.4.2 Inconsistencies Across Regions

Another subgroup analysis that gave the FDA and its Advisory Committee a hard time was presented as part of the New Drug Application (NDA) of ticagrelor. The platelet inhibition and clinical outcomes (PLATO) trial revealed a significant benefit of ticagrelor over clopidogrel in terms of the composite endpoint of cardiovascular death, myocardial infarction or stroke at one year in patients with acute coronary symptoms [hazard ratio 0.84, 95% CI (0.77, 0.92), $p < 0.001$] (Wallentin et al., 2009). Much discussion was generated by the finding that ticagrelor offered no benefit over clopidogrel in the United States (Table 1.5).

A similar situation occurred earlier in 2001 for the MERIT-HF[5] where a post hoc subgroup analysis showed a mortality hazard ratio of 1.05 (95% CI (0.71, 1.56)) for the United States and 0.55 (0.43, 0.70) for all other countries combined and a significant quantitative interaction ($p = 0.003$) (Wedel et al., 2001).

In search for an explanation of the PLATO results, the differing aspirin (ASA) dose between the regions was identified as a potential cause by the sponsor. Specifically, a higher maintenance dose of aspirin was associated with relatively unfavorable outcomes with tigacrelor in both US and non-US patients while the hazard ratios for low-dose aspirin look similar, however with a much lower sample size in the United States as compared to the non-US region (see Table 1.5).

---

[5]MERIT-HF = metoprolol controlled release randomized intervention trial in heart failure

Table 1.5 PLATO results overall and by region and ASA dose (mg)

Subgroup	Tigacrelor		Clopidogrel		HR (95% CI)
	N	Events	N	Events	
All	9333	864	0291	1014	0.84 (0.77, 0.92)
US	707	84	706	67	1.27 (0.92, 1.75)
Non-US	8626	780	8585	947	0.81 (0.74, 0.90)
ASA ≥ 300	464	68	492	50	1.45 (1.01, 2.09)
100 < ASA < 300	525	64	527	65	0.99 (0.70, 1.40)
ASA ≤ 100	7733	565	7706	723	0.77 (0.69, 0.86)

https://www.accessdata.fda.govdrugsatfda_docs/label/2015/022433s015lbl.pdf

22 Some History of Subgroup Analysis

The other potential explanation was a difference in monitoring among regions. It seems hard, however, to imagine how this should have affected mortality. At the end of the day, ticagrelor was approved in the United States; however, the lack of efficacy in the US and the potential impact of the aspirin dose had to be included in the label (Gaglia and Waksman, 2011). Buyse and Marschner (2011) provided further support of no variation in treatment effect beyond chance.

It would have been interesting to see how the PMDA (Pharmaceuticals and Medical Devices Agency), the Japanese health authority, would have reacted if the results had occurred in Japan instead of the United States. Following their guidelines (MHLW, 2007), they only accept the results of an international trial for drug approval if the observed treatment effect in Japan is at least half of the overall study effect estimate or if all regional effects are less than 0 (if a reduction of an endpoint constitutes a success). Applying either criterion, tigacrelor may have failed in Japan.

1.4.3 Detecting Non-responders

An example where post hoc subgroup analyses led to product label changes resulting in restrictions of the patient population is cetuximab. The drug got approval for epidermal growth factor receptor (EGFR) expressing metastatic colorectal cancer in 2004. However, retrospective subgroup analyses suggested a lack of efficacy in patients with

Table 1.6 Results for the PLATO trial by ASA dose within region

Region	ASA dose (mg)	Tigacrelor		Clopidogrel		HR (95% CI)
		N	Events	N	Events	
US	≥ 300	324	40	352	27	1.62 (0.99, 2.64)
	(100, 300)	22	2	16	2	—
	≤ 100	284	19	263	24	0.73 (0.40, 1.33)
Non-US	≥ 300	140	28	140	23	1.23 (0.71, 2.14)
	(100, 300)	503	62	511	63	1.00 (0.71, 1.42)
	≤ 100	7449	546	7443	699	0.78 (0.69, 0.87)

https://www.accessdata.fda.govdrugsatfda_docs/label/2015/022433s015lbl.pdf

metastatic disease whose tumors have KRAS[6] mutations. KRAS, an essential component of the EGFR signaling cascade, can acquire mutations that render EGFR inhibitors ineffective.

We summarize the results of one of the studies (Jonker et al., 2007) that was analyzed further in Karapetis et al. (2008) after the observation of resistance to cetuximab with a 50% progression rate at the first assessment of disease progression and a median progression-free survival that did not differ between the groups (1.8 months in the supportive-care group versus 1.9 months in the cetuximab group). The disease was stable or responded to therapy in only 39.4% of the patients in the cetuximab group, a result indicating a need for predictive biomarkers to identify patients who could benefit from such treatment (Jonker et al., 2007).

Tumor samples obtained from 394 of 572 patients were analyzed to look for activating mutations of the K-ras gene. Of the tumors evaluated, 42.3% in the supportive care group and 40.9% in the cetuximab group had at least one mutation. The interaction of K-ras mutation status with overall survival and progression-free survival was significant with $p = 0.01$ and $p < 0.001$, respectively, indicating an association between these variables and genetic status. The main results of the analysis are shown in Table 1.7. The subgroup analyses eventually led to a labeling

[6]v-Ki-ras2 Kirsten rat sarcoma viral oncogene homolog

Table 1.7 Median (progression-free) survival and hazard ratios

K-ras	Survival (months)			PFS (months)		
	Cet	SC	HR (95% CI)	Cet	SC	HR (95% CI)
Mutation	4.5	4.6	0.98 (0.70, 1.37)	1.8	1.8	0.99 (0.73, 1.35)
Wild type	9.5	4.8	0.55 (0.41, 0.74)	3.7	1.9	0.40 (0.30, 0.54)

PFS = progression-free survival, Cet = cetuximab, SC = supportive care, HR = hazard ratio, CI = confidence interval. Source: (Karapetis et al., 2008)

revision by FDA in 2009: "Retrospective subset analyses of metastatic or advanced colorectal cancer trials have not shown a treatment benefit for Erbitux in patients whose tumors had KRAS mutations in codon 12 or 13. Use of Erbitux is not recommended for the treatment of colorectal cancer with these mutations."[7]

1.4.4 In Search for Benefit

Another interesting debate on the interpretation of the overall study result and subgroup analyses took place in the Journal of Clinical Epidemiology in 2010. The authors of the CAPRIE[8] study (CAPRIE Steering Committee, 1996) felt annoyed by the, in their opinion, inconsistent assessments of two agencies, the British National Institute for Health and Clinical Excellence (NICE) and the German Institute for Quality and Effiency in Healthcare (IQWiQ) (Hasford et al., 2010).

CAPRIE compared the use of clopidogrel versus aspirin in the secondary prevention of vascular events (myocardial infarction (MI), ischemic stroke (IS), or vascular death) in patients with atherothrombosis as diagnosed by recent MI, recent stroke, or symptomatic peripheral arterial disease (PAD). The intention-to-treat (ITT) analysis of 19 185 patients showed an annual 5.32%

---

[7] https://www.accessdata.fda.gov/drugsatfda_docs/label/2009/125084s167lbl.pdf

[8] CAPRIE = Clopidogrel versus aspirin in patients at risk of ischemic events

risk of IS, MI, or vascular death under clopidogrel compared with 5.83% under aspirin, yielding a statistically significant ($p = 0.043$) relative risk reduction of 8.7% in favor of clopidogrel (95% confidence interval 0.3 to 16.5).

The study protocol considered a stratified randomization and sample size planning accounting for different event rates for MI, stroke or PAD. The publication contained an analysis for each of these subgroups summarized as in Table 1.8 and using a forest plot as shown in Figure 1.1. A treatment by subgroup interaction test was statistically significant ($p = 0.042$). Despite that, FDA approved clopidogrel for the entire study population in 1997 mentioning in their report that it is not clear whether the difference is real or a chance occurrence. In a meta-analysis, the agency discovered the strongest results of aspirin in patients with recent MI and lower efficacy in other subgroups (FDA, 1997). IQWiQ, however, considered these subgroups as preplanned and

Table 1.8 Relative risk reduction with 95% confidence interval (CI) by subgroup and overall in CAPRIE study

Subgroup	RRR(%)	95% CI	p-value
Stroke	7.3	(−5.7, 18.7)	0.26
MI	−3.7	(−22.1, 12.0)	0.66
PAD	23.8	(8.9, 36.2)	0.0028
All	8.7	(0.3, 16.5)	0.043

28 Some History of Subgroup Analysis

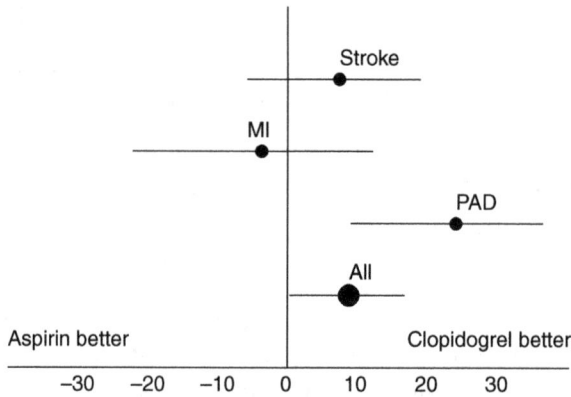

Figure 1.1 Relative risk reduction with 95% confidence intervals by subgroup and overall in CAPRIE study.

acknowledged an additional benefit of clopidogrel exclusively for the PAD subgroup because of heterogeneity of results (Bender et al., 2010).

In the view of Hasford et al. (2010), NICE concluded with respect to efficacy in accordance with the primary analysis of the overall population. However, it considered the balance between clinical effectiveness and cost-effectiveness not to justify a replacement of aspirin by clopidogrel to prevent vascular events. Therefore, NICE's and IQWiQ's conclusions were not that far apart since both agencies stated that the data do not show consistent benefit of clopidogrel but rather non-inferiority. In the last editorial on the topic (Hasford et al., 2011) the opponents concluded that "Standards for subgroup analyses are needed?—we could not agree more."

1.5 CONCLUDING REMARKS

This chapter has presented a selection of the good, the bad, and the ugly subgroup analyses from the past. In those cases that were part of submissions, regulatory agencies had to make a decision on how the results from subgroups affect the label of the compound. It becomes obvious from this account that there is at times a fine line between the reasonable and the ridiculous. Unfortunately, the ridiculous is not always as obvious as the star-sign determined subgroups in the ISIS–2 study.

In many cases, a biological rationale is helpful to "separate the wheat from the chaff." However, preferably the rationale should be available at the planning stage and not post hoc, otherwise it may become triggered by suggestive results. In any case, some form of replication of results should occur to assess credibility of subgroup findings. Comparing results with other research and searching for corroboration should be undertaken. For results with a big impact replication may be the action of choice or, as Rothwell (2005) has put it: the best test of the validity of subgroup analyses is not significance but replication.

2

Objectives and Current Practice of Subgroup Analyses

> *This leads directly to a related criticism of the present controlled trial – that it does not tell the doctor what he wants to know. It may be so constituted as to show without any doubt that treatment A is on the average better than treatment B. On the other hand, that result does not answer the practicing doctor's question – what is the most likely outcome when this drug is given to a particular patient? (Bradford Hill, 1966)*
>
> Sir Austin Bradford Hill (1897–1991)

2.1 INTRODUCTION

The topic of subgroup analyses has primarily two aspects: why would we embark into them in the first place, i.e. what are their objectives, and what tools are at our disposals to address the objectives. Furthermore, over time a fair amount of terminology and definitions have arisen to characterize different types of subgroups. Another topic is the currently most used subgroup analyses and how analyses and results are reported in medical journals.

2.2 OBJECTIVES OF SUBGROUP ANALYSES

The most straightforward aim of subgroup analyses is to *estimate* parameters related to treatment effects in predefined subgroups. In this situation, accurate (unbiased) estimation is possible; however, estimators may lack precision because of the reduced sample size of a subset as compared to the full data. In Chapter 5 it will be shown how the precision of estimators can be improved (at the expense of some bias) by applying hierarchical modeling to the data.

A second objective constitutes *selection* or identification of subsets of individuals in whom treatment effects differ from the overall population. For example, a drug may have moderate efficacy in the overall study population but a much better efficacy in a subset of subjects and none in others. The selection of the former subset is often based on large effect estimates or significant test results, which can lead to over-optimistic effect estimators in the selected group. Thus methods to identify subsets of high efficacy should be complemented with methods that correct for selection bias. One method to achieve this aim is presented in Chapter 6.

An objective in between estimation and selection is *verifying the consistency* of the treatment effect across subgroups in a more formal way than just looking at individual group estimates. This objective is advocated for example in a European Subgroup Analysis Guideline (EMA, 2019). One option to address this are interaction tests, which are discussed in Section 2.5.

Another objective could be to *predict* the benefit from a specific treatment over a reference or placebo for a future individual given his biomarker data. In this case, one would also like to know the prediction error of the prediction. This objective is likely addressing best Sir Bradford Hill's request (Bradford Hill, 1966) stated at the beginning of this chapter and is taken on in Chapters 7 and 8.

Eventually the confirmatory *testing* of treatment effects in subgroups can be an objective. This results in higher variability of test statistics, which may be compensated for by larger effects in some subgroups. Furthermore, multiplicity issues may have to be considered, potentially reducing the power of the tests. Confirmatory testing comes most often into the game when the number of subgroups is limited.

To be able to define or select subgroups, information beyond treatment and results is needed for the individuals in a trial. Patient characteristics or biomarkers (like age, disease history or severity, genetic information, etc.), called covariables or covariates in statistical language, are used to define subgroups. Often, these variables are incorporated into a statistical model describing the relationship between treatment, biomarkers and results. An overview of how covariates can be used to characterize subgroups and achieve the objectives above is given in Chapter 4.

2.3 DEFINITIONS AROUND SUBGROUPS

Following Yusuf et al. (1991), a *proper subgroup* in a clinical trial is a group of patients characterized by a common set of baseline (pre-treatment) covariates like:

- Inherent patient characteristics that cannot be affected by treatment like age, sex, ethnicity, genetic constellation.
- Disease characteristics, e.g. type or severity, assessed before the start of treatment.

An *improper subgroup* in a clinical trial is a group of patients characterized by variables measured post-baseline (after the start of interventions) that are potentially affected by treatment like

Definitions Around Subgroups

compliance to study protocol, completion of study, non-response, or need for rescue medication.

Subgroups are *predefined* or *pre-specified* if they are identified before the start of study or in masked trials at least before unblinding of the treatment information. This approach has a high degree of credibility since it offers transparency about what is intended and allows for prospective planning of analyses. Having to think rigorously about potential subgroups beforehand may also limit the number of envisaged subgroups.

Nevertheless it has to be admitted that not all potentially relevant subgroups can be thought of beforehand since surprises are an essential part of research. In such cases it may be required to define subgroups *post-hoc* since they are selected after having analyzed the data. These analyses have clearly a much lower level of credibility, because, to quote Senn and Harrell (1997), the equivalent in horse racing would be, rather than betting on a named horse, to write "first past the post" on the betting slip and collect the winnings, whatever the results. This criticism applies specifically when an attempt is made to salvage a trial with overall unsatisfying results by searching subgroups with a positive effect.

However, when unexpected safety results occur there is likely no alternative to follow-up regardless of pre-specification. In any case subgroups to be analyzed should be documented in the protocol to be able to discern the pre-defined and the post-hoc defined ones in the report or the publication.

Subgroups are called *prognostic* if the course of the disease differs between subgroups regardless of treatment. Subgroups are *predictive* for a specific treatment if its effect differs between subgroups. In parallel group trials, prognostic effects relate to control treatment and predictive effects to the test or experimental treatment.

A differential subgroup effect of test over control is called a *quantitative interaction* if a treatment is truly beneficial (or harmful) in all subgroups, but the magnitude of effect varies. A differential subgroup effect is called a *qualitative interaction* if treatment is truly beneficial in some and truly harmful in other subgroups.

Assume that subgroups can be characterized by a set of binary baseline covariates $X_1, \ldots, X_K$. A *k-variate subgroup* is defined in terms of k covariates:

$$S_{i_1, \ldots, i_k}(x_{i_1}, \ldots, x_{i_k}) = \left\{ \begin{array}{l} \text{all subjects with } X_{i_l} = x_{i_l} \\ \text{for all } l = 1, \ldots, k \end{array} \right\}.$$

For $k = K$, all subgroups are non-overlapping while if $k < K$, k-variate subgroups can overlap, i.e., one individual can belong to several subgroups. The number of potential k-variate subgroups is $\binom{K}{k} 2^k$ which results in $2K$ for $k = 1$ and 2^K for $k = K$. A large number of subgroups leads to a large number of *small* subgroups.

A *univariate subgroup* is defined in terms of a single covariate:

$$S_k(x) = \{\text{all subjects with } X_k = x\}, \quad x = 0, 1.$$

These subgroups are most commonly addressed in the demography or subjects disposition reporting of clinical trials. Univariate subgroup treatment effect estimators $\hat{\theta}(x_k)$ can be obtained from multivariate subgroup effects $\hat{\theta}(\mathbf{x})$ as follows (Varadhan and Wang, 2016):

$$\hat{\theta}(x_k) = \sum_{\mathbf{x}} \hat{\theta}(\mathbf{x}) \Pr[\mathbf{X}_{\neq k} = \mathbf{x}_{\neq k} | X_x = x_k].$$

($\mathbf{X}_{\neq k}$ denotes the vector of covariates without the k-th variable.) Since K-variate effect estimators are independent one obtains

$$V[\hat{\theta}(x_k)] = \sum_{\mathbf{x}} \Pr[\mathbf{X}_{\neq k} = \mathbf{x}_{\neq k} | X_x = x_k]^2 V[\hat{\theta}(\mathbf{X})].$$

2.4 CONFOUNDING

Since we consider mainly randomized studies, the assigned treatment T is independent of any other baseline covariate. What can happen if this condition is not satisfied is shown in Section 3.6. However, if $X_1, \ldots, X_K$ are correlated, k-variate subgroups may be confounded with the following consequences:

- If one of two positively correlated covariates is an effect modifier, the other can be identified as predictive.
- If two covariates are negatively correlated and both are effect modifiers, their marginal effects can cancel.

How relevant is confounding? According to VanderWeele and Knol (2011), if the question of interest is to assess whether an effect varies across strata of a covariate (so-called "effect heterogeneity"), confounding is not relevant and does not need to be controlled for. However, if one intends to attribute the differences in treatment effect to a specific covariate (so-called "causal interaction") to intervene for maximization of a treatment effect, confounding is relevant and must be controlled for.

Stratifying randomization with regard to covariates does not suffice to control for confounding covariates; it simply increases the probability that comparable numbers of subjects receiving treatment and control would be included in each stratum. Only if randomization of a covariate would be possible, confounding would be eliminated for this variable (similarly to treatment assignment).

Confounding can also be counteracted by assigning standardization weights to data (Varadhan and Wang, 2014):

$$w_k(\mathbf{x}) = \frac{\Pr[X_k = x_k]}{\Pr[X_k = x_k | \mathbf{X}_{\neq k} = \mathbf{x}_{\neq k}]}.$$

Unfortunately, weights can become large for small subgroups (i.e. for large K) resulting in unstable estimates w_k.

2.5 TWO TYPES OF SUBGROUP ANALYSES

There are basically two ways in which subgroup effects are analyzed most of the time. The first is to compare test and control treatment within each subgroup. Although this approach is fairly straightforward, the results may be difficult to interpret, since it does not answer the question of a differential effect between subgroups.

A situation where the difficulties in interpretation become apparent is depicted in Figure 2.1. In this example it is assumed that the overall analysis of the data yields a p-value of 0.01. For $0 \leq q \leq 1$, the data are then arbitrarily split into two subgroups comprising $100q\%$ and $100(1-q)\%$ of

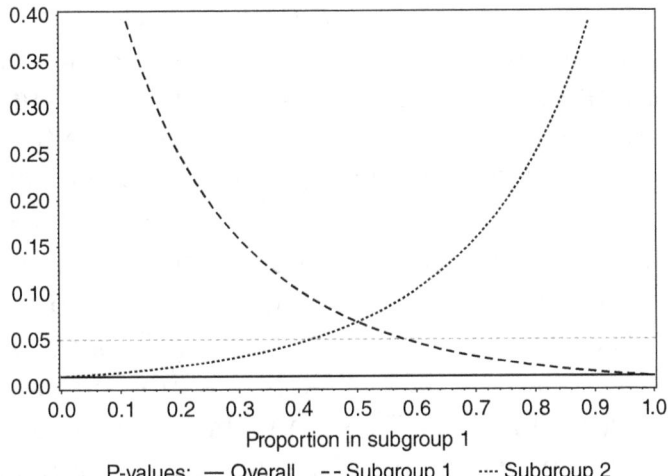

Figure 2.1 P-values in subgroups if point estimates in subgroups are identical for an overall p-value of 0.01.

the data, respectively. If the average effect in these subgroups is the same, the p-values for the within subgroup comparisons depend entirely on q. For $q \leq 0.4$, the p-value from a comparison in subgroup 2 is below 0.05, while the p-value from subgroup 1 always exceeds 0.05. This relationship holds for $q \geq 0.4$ with subgroups interchanged. Hence despite equal effect estimators only one subgroup can become significant. This may lead to the conclusion that there is an effect in one subgroup but not in the other one in the absence of a differential effect.

Alternatively, one can analyze treatment by subgroup interactions, which would answer the question of heterogeneity directly (Assmann et al., 2000). This approach may require data modeling to define interactions properly.

Brookes et al. (2001) performed a simulation study to compare false positive subgroup findings from interaction tests and from tests within subgroups. For what they call the simplest case they simulated 100 000 datasets consisting of normally distributed variables with two subgroups, completely balanced treatment assignment and zero overall and subgroup effects. In the approximately 95% of datasets correctly finding no overall treatment effect exactly one subgroup was significant in about 7%. Among the 5% of datasets with an incorrectly significant overall treatment effect, a large percentage of the analyses – up to 64% – found a treatment effect in one subgroup only (see Table 2.1). The false positive findings

Table 2.1 Percentage of false positive subgroup findings conditional on overall effect and overall significance (Brookes et al., 2001, 2004)

Overall effect	Overall effect significant at 5%	Only one within subgroup effect significant at 5%
Yes	Yes	≈ 57%
	No	≈ 21%
No	Yes	≈ 64%
	No	≈ 7%

of an interaction test are about 5% regardless of overall significance.

Data were also simulated with an overall treatment effect but no differential subgroup effects. We report the findings for a sample size corresponding to 80% overall power. In datasets with a correct significant overall effect, one subgroup only became significant in about 57%, neither subgroup in about 13% of the simulations. In the case of a false-negative overall finding, only one subgroup was significant in about 21% of the simulations (see Table 2.1). There are clear lessons to be learned from this investigation:

- Concluding a subgroup effect in the case of a significant result in just one subgroup results in a false positive rate exceeding 5%.
- The chance of obtaining a significant result in exactly one subgroup in an overall non-significant trial ranges between 7% and 21% in the absence of any subgroup effect.

- On the other hand if the overall test is significant, the chance to detect a difference in exactly one subgroup is between 57% and 64% in the absence of a subgroup effect.
- The risk to incorrectly conclude an effect in just one subgroup in an overall positive trial is much larger than in an overall negative trial.
- The chance to salvage an overall non-significant trial by a subgroup analysis in the absence of subgroup effects is much lower than the chance to falsely detect a subgroup effect in an overall positive trial.

As a consequence of the last bullet point, regulators should be more afraid of falsely detecting heterogeneities of the data in the case of an overall significant effect than about false positive subgroup effects in an overall non-significantly different comparison. Currently it seems to be the other way round (see EMA (2019)).

The interaction test has clear advantages in terms of interpretation; however, it has power issues. Generally it has the same power as the overall test if the interaction effect is twice the overall effect while an interaction effect of the same magnitude as the overall effect can be detected with a power of 29% for an overall power of 80%. (Brookes et al., 2001).

The dilemma of within and between subgroup analyses was succinctly summarized in Yusuf et al. (1991): "Generally, trials adequate for detecting an overall treatment effect cannot be expected to detect effects within subgroups and are very unlikely to detect interactions."

2.6 REPORTING OF SUBGROUPS

Statements in the publication of clinical trials like "We explored analyses of numerous other subgroups to assess the effect of baseline prognostic factors or coexisting conditions on the treatment effect but found no evidence of nominal significance for any biologically likely factor" (Lees et al., 2006) are not uncommon. An analysis of completeness and quality of subgroup analyses reported in the New England Journal of Medicine between July 1, 2005 through June 30, 2006, conducted in Wang et al. (2007) can be summarized as follows:

- 59 studies reported subgroup analyses that were mentioned in the "methods" section for 21 trials (36%), in the "results" section for 57 trials (97%), and in the "discussion" for 37 trials (63%).
- The number of subgroup analyses conducted was generally unclear.
- In 40 trials (68%), it was unclear whether any of the subgroup analyses were pre-specified or not.
- Interaction tests were used to assess heterogeneity of treatment effects for all subgroups in 16 trials (27%), for some but not all in 11 trials (19%) and never in 32 trials (54%).

According to Gabler et al. (2016) and Fan et al. (2019), the situation has not improved much since then. These authors conclude that justification or rationale for subgroup analyses were only rarely provided in study protocols or reports.

The Consolidated Standards of Reporting Trials (CONSORT) (Schulz et al., 2010) provide guidance for reporting all randomized controlled trials focusing on individually randomized, two group, parallel trials (other designs are covered in extensions). They contain also some advice on the reporting of subgroups as summarized in Table 2.2.

Table 2.2 Reporting of subgroups as proposed by CONSORT 2010

Topic	#	Checklist item
Statistical methods	12b	Methods for additional analyses, such as **subgroup** and adjusted analyses
Ancillary analyses	18	Results of any other analyses performed, including **subgroup** and adjusted analyses, distinguishing **pre-specified from exploratory**
Limitations	20	Trial limitations, addressing sources of **potential bias**, **imprecision**, and, if relevant, **multiplicity** of analyses

2.7 CONCLUDING REMARKS

This chapter has provided a systematic account of current practice of subgroup analyses – objectives, definitions, analysis and reporting. The next chapter will summarize the potential pitfalls of subgroup analyses before the rest of the book focuses on analyses of data including a moderate number of pre-defined proper subgroups, i.e. subgroups defined by baseline covariates. Analyses are meant to be exploratory, either by estimation of subgroup effects, selecting subgroups or predicting effects. Confirmatory subgroup analyses are not within the scope of this book. For further reading on this topic we refer to Alosh et al. (2015, 2017) and Ondra et al. (2016).

3

Pitfalls of Subgroup Analyses

> *It was the best of times, it was the worst of times, it was the age of wisdom, it was the age of foolishness, it was the epoch of belief, it was the epoch of incredulity.*
>
> Charles Dickens (1812-1870)—A Tale of Two Cities

3.1 INTRODUCTION

From Chapter 1 it is obvious that – regardless of one's attitude towards subgroup analyses – there are some potential pitfalls of subgroup analyses requiring attention. In the following a more systematic account of these fallacies will be given. An underlying theme in the discussion of the present chapter is that often an observed effect can be attributed to chance rather than to a systematic effect.

Most clinical trials are designed for an assessment of an overall or average treatment effect (ATE). As a consequence, comparisons within or between subgroups, i.e. by means of interactions, will be less informative because of the smaller sample sizes leading to false-negative assessments. At the same time, the high number of comparisons increases the risk of false-positive decisions. If multiplicity is accounted for, the false-negative rate will increase further. One way out is to run larger clinical trials focusing on a small number of subgroups. As a consequence, meaningful subgroup analyses could lead to larger and not necessarily to smaller studies.

3.2 EXTREME EFFECT ESTIMATES

Wainer and Zwerling (2006) report on a study of the incidence of kidney cancer in the 3141 counties of the United States. The study revealed that the counties in which the incidence of kidney cancer is lowest are mostly rural, sparsely populated, and located in traditionally Republican states in the Midwest, the South, and the West. What conclusions can be drawn from this statement?

Very likely, most people would reject the idea that Republican politics protects against cancer and focus on the fact that the counties with low incidence are mostly rural and infer this to the clean living of the rural lifestyle – no air or water pollution, and access to fresh food.

When considering the counties in which the incidence of kidney cancer is highest one finds that they tend to be mostly rural, sparsely populated, and located in traditionally Republican states in the Midwest, the South, and the West. The high rates could be directly related to the poverty of the rural lifestyle – no access to good medical care, a high-fat diet, and too much alcohol and tobacco.

Something is wrong here: the rural lifestyle cannot explain both very high and very low incidences. A more plausible explanation is simply – chance: rural areas are less populated than other areas and extreme outcomes are most likely to be found in sparsely populated counties. Kahneman (2012) calls this the "law of small numbers."

Looking at clinical trials, subgroups have smaller sample sizes than the overall patient population under investigation. This does not only imply a reduction of power to detect differences within or between subgroups, but also an increased risk of observing extreme effect estimates. The latter can easily be quantified as follows.

Let $Y_1, \ldots, Y_N$ be independent normally distributed variables with zero mean and unit variance.

Then the arithmetic mean $\overline{Y} = \sum_{n=1}^{N} Y_n/N$ is also normally distributed with zero mean but variance $1/N$. If Φ denotes the cdf of a standard normal variable it follows that

$$\Pr[|\overline{Y}| \geq c] = \Pr[\overline{Y} \geq c] + \Pr[\overline{Y} \leq -c]$$
$$= 1 - \Phi(c\sqrt{N}) + \Phi(-c\sqrt{N})$$
$$= 2(1 - \Phi(c\sqrt{N})).$$

Table 3.1 displays this probability for $c = 0.2$ and $N = 10, \ldots, 100$. Furthermore, if a subgroup is chosen based on the largest effect estimate, as is often the case, smaller subgroups have a greater chance to be selected than larger ones even if the the within subgroup effects are the same.

Table 3.1 Probability of large effect estimates.

N	$\Pr[|\overline{Y}| \geq 0.2]$
10	0.52709
20	0.37109
30	0.27332
40	0.20590
50	0.15730
60	0.12134
70	0.09426
80	0.07364
90	0.05778
100	0.04550

$\overline{Y}$ is the average of N independent standard normal variables.

3.3 SELECTION BIAS

Consider the following situation: a pharmaceutical company intends to license in a drug for the treatment of a specific condition. The results of a clinical trial conducted by a start-up look better than those of competitors' compounds available. After the successful deal, the company repeats the trial to confirm the results, but the new results do not live up to the expectations created by the first trial. Has the company been betrayed by faked data? Or have they been overoptimistic when looking at the original results?

To answer this question consider the following task: from two sets of normally distributed data select the one with the largest mean and estimate the maximum of the means. Obviously one would select the dataset with the largest arithmetic mean and would use it as an estimator of the maximum of means. Unfortunately, this procedure would result in an upwards bias, i.e. the estimate obtained would likely be too optimistic, as in the license deal situation. .

Let the data be distributed as $N(\theta_t, 1)$, $t = 0, 1$, and let $\overline{Y}_t$ be the corresponding arithmetic means and $\overline{Y}_{(0)} \leq \overline{Y}_{(1)}$ the order statistics. Let n_t denote the respective sample sizes and Let $\tau^2 = 1/n_0 + 1/n_1$. Then the selection bias of $\overline{Y}_{(1)}$ relative to $\max(\theta_0, \theta_1)$ is given by (Venter, 1988):

$$\tau\phi(|\theta_1 - \theta_0|/\tau)$$

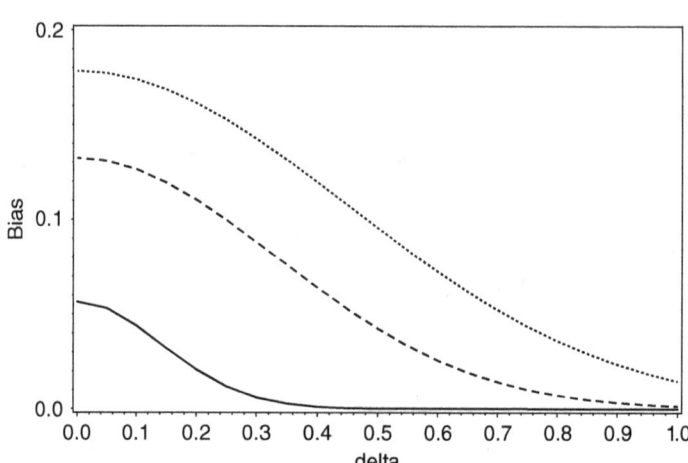

Figure 3.1 Bias of the estimator of the maximum of two means of standard normal data as a function of sample size ($n = (n_0, n_1)$) and mean difference δ.

where ϕ denotes the pdf of a standard normal variable. As can be seen, the bias depends on the unknown parameters, is largest ($=\tau/\sqrt{2\pi}$) for $\delta = \theta_0 - \theta_1 = 0$ and disappears for large $\min(n_0, n_1)$ (see Figure 3.1). In fact there is no unbiased estimator of the maximum of the means of normal distributions (Cohen and Sackrowitz, 1989; Stallard et al., 2008).

The latter is not good news. Considering the predominance of maximum likelihood estimators, which are (asymptotically) normally distributed (Wald, 1943), selecting the group with maximum estimate may lead to biased estimators that cannot be completely adjusted.

There are distributions for which unbiased estimators of the maximum exist. For exponentially distributed data $Y_{tn} \sim \exp(1/\theta_t)$, $n = 1, \ldots, N$,

$$\overline{Y}_{(1)}\{1 - [\overline{Y}_{(0)}/\overline{Y}_{(1)}]^n\}$$

is an unbiased estimator of $\max(\theta_0, \theta_1)$ (Vallaisamy and Sharma, 1988). In Chapter 6 we consider a generic way to reduce bias after selection.

3.4 REVERSAL OF EFFECTS

Drug regulating agencies, in particular, are interested in knowing whether an overall treatment effect is consistent across subgroups (FDA, 1988; EMA, 2019). This raises the question of how often it can happen by chance alone that effect estimates are positive in some subgroups and negative in others under consistent treatment effects. An assessment of this question is important in the interpretation of clinical trials, as shown by the controversies over the CAPRIE, PLATO and TAYLORx results discussed in Chapter 1.

Li et al. (2007) investigated the probability of observing negative subgroup results when the treatment effect is positive and homogeneous across all subgroups in the setting of normally distributed outcomes. Let Y_t represent the measurements of a patient receiving treatment t ($t = 0, 1$). Assume that Y_t is normally distributed with mean θ_t and variance σ^2. Let $\delta = \theta_1 - \theta_0$,

Pitfalls of Subgroup Analyses

where $\delta < 0$ represents a more desirable outcome. Let $2N$ be the number of subjects in the trial, divided equally between the treatment groups, and let $N_{t1}, \ldots, N_{tK}$ denote the number of subjects in subgroup k ($k = 1, \ldots, K$) assigned to treatment t.

The treatment effect in subgroup k is estimated by the observed mean difference D_k between the N_{1k} subjects on treatment 1 and the N_{0k} subjects on treatment 0. Then D_k is normally distributed with mean $\delta < 0$ and variance $\sigma^2 N_k/(N_{0k}N_{1k})$, where $N_k = N_{0k} + N_{1k}$. If D_k is obtained from mutually exclusive subgroups (like for example centers, regions, disease severity, etc.) they are independent. The probability P_{1K} of observing at least one positive D_k is

$$P_{1K} = 1 - \prod_{k=1}^{K} \Pr[D_k \leq 0]$$

$$= 1 - \prod_{k=1}^{K} \Phi\left(-\frac{\delta}{\sigma}\sqrt{\frac{N_{0k}N_{1k}}{N_k}}\right). \quad (3.1)$$

From Equation 3.1 it can be seen that the following factors affect the probability of at least one positive subgroup result:

- P_{1K} decreases if the effect increases, i.e. $\delta/\sigma < 0$ decreases.
- When the number of subgroups is fixed, P_{1K} decreases as the number of subjects increases.
- When other factors are fixed, P_{1K} is minimized if the treatment assignment is balanced in all

subgroups. In practice, this can be achieved by stratified randomization.

- When other factors are fixed and treatment assignment is balanced in all subgroups, P_{1K} is minimized if all subgroups are equally represented.
- Assuming a fixed sample size and equally represented subgroups, P_{1K} increases with the number of subgroups.

A numerical illustration is provided in Table 3.2 for an homogeneous treatment effect size of -0.5. Sample sizes were chosen so that the study provided an 80% or 90% power to detect this effect size. The probability for at least one positive outcome is fairly substantial. Note that the figures are produced under the assumption of mutually

Table 3.2 Probability of observing at least one positive subgroup result when the effect size is -0.5 in all three subgroups (Li et al., 2007)

Proportion of subgroups	Sample size per group	
	64 (80% power)	86 (90% power)
(0.33, 0.33, 0.33)	14.6	8.5
(0.2, 0.6, 0.2)	20.7	14.2
(0.1, 0.8, 0.1)	34.0	27.9
(0.2, 0.2, 0.2, 0.2, 0.2)	41.9	30.9
(0.1, 0.2, 0.2, 0.4, 0.1)	48.6	38.9
(0.1, 0.1, 0.1, 0.1, 0.6)	56.6	48.1

exclusive subgroups. They get smaller if subjects belong to more than one subgroup (e.g., male subjects with severe disease). For details see Li et al. (2007). Quan et al. (2010) thought about assessing the consistency of treatment effects in multi-regional clinical trials and came up with five potential consistency criteria, two in terms of treatment effect estimates and three in terms of hypotheses testing:

1. Achieving in each region a specified proportion of the observed overall effect.
2. Observing region effects that exceed a pre-specified effect size in all regions.
3. Demonstrating that all region effects exceed a proportion of the overall effect.
4. Absence of significant treatment-by-region interaction.
5. Lack of significant difference for any regions from the overall.

Criteria 1 and 2 refer to conditions that have to hold for all regions. The third criterion is the testing analogue to criterion 1. The chance that one of these criteria will be fulfilled under consistency will always be lower than the power for detecting an overall effect. This confirms the finding that effect estimate reversals have a fair change to occur. Criteria 4 and 5 are looking for the absence of significance, which does of course not imply the absence of an interaction or a difference.

3.5 REGRESSION TO THE MEAN

A regression effect is the tendency of extreme values to move closer to the mean when measured a second time. Regression to the mean was discovered by Sir Francis Galton, published in 1886 under the title "Regression towards mediocrity in hereditary stature." He reports measurements of size in successive generations of seeds and comparisons of the height of children to the height of their parents. Galton realized that the offspring tended to be smaller than the parents if the latter were large, and to be larger than parents if the latter were small. For an appreciation of Galton's work see Senn (2011).

Consider now a study where patients get their blood pressure measured before and after treatment to investigate whether therapy lowers it. Typically, only patients with high blood pressure are admitted into such a study. Their blood pressure will tend to decrease, on average, during the trial regardless of the efficacy of treatment provided. This can be seen as follows.

Let X, Y denote two normally distributed variables with mean μ, standard deviation σ and correlation $-1 \leq \rho \leq 1$. Then

$$E[Y|X = x] = \mu + \rho(x - \mu)$$

If $|\rho| < 1$ it follows that

$$|E[Y|X = x] - \mu| < |x - \mu|. \qquad (3.2)$$

Identifying X with the baseline and Y with the post-baseline measurement, the conditional expectation of the post-baseline value is closer to the mean μ than the baseline value, though the treatment effect is zero since the distribution of Y and X are identical. The weaker the correlation between the two variables, the stronger this shrinkage effect is. Equation (3.2) is the mathematical formulation of regression to the mean. In the case $0 < \rho < 1$, we obtain

$$E[Y|X = x] < x, \quad \text{if } x > \mu$$
$$E[Y|X = x] > x, \quad \text{if } x < \mu$$

suggesting an on average reduction in the post-baseline value if the baseline value is above the mean. Recall, however, that there is no difference in the means of the entire population. The difference in the subsets is due to the selection process only. In drug development, this scenario is a major reason for having a control group included in clinical trials (patients not receiving the treatment of interest, but otherwise undergoing exactly the same selection and clinical procedures). The control group provides a reference against which the treatment group(s) of interest can be compared, the only difference being the treatment effect itself.

What can be done in the absence of a control group to disentangle the regression to the mean effect and the net treatment effect? Naranjo and McKean (2001) propose a dual effects model for normally distributed variables. A flexible approach allowing for modeling the outcome measurement is described in Krause and Pinheiro (2007). We briefly explain the latter for the bivariate normal situation. First one obtains estimates $\overline{X}$, $\overline{Y}$, $\hat{\sigma}_X^2$, $\hat{\sigma}_Y^2$, $\hat{\sigma}_{XY}$ for the means, variances and covariances of the variables X and Y from the full dataset. A paired t-test on the difference of the baseline and post-baseline measurement provides a p-value p_{obs}.

Next, one estimates the means and variances of X and Y under the assumption of equal distributions or no change by

$$\tilde{X} = \tilde{Y} = (\overline{X} + \overline{Y})/2$$
$$\tilde{\sigma}_X^2 = \tilde{\sigma}_Y^2 = (\hat{\sigma}_X^2 + \hat{\sigma}_Y^2)/2.$$

Eventually one simulates M datasets from this null model, each with the same number of observations as the original data after having discarded all data points with too small values of X. Conducting a paired t-test for each dataset results in p-values p_m, $m = 1, \ldots, M$, given by

$$p_{\text{adj}} = \frac{1}{M} \sum_{m=1}^{M} I(p_m \leq p_{\text{obs}})$$

where I denotes the indicator function with $I(A) = 1$ if A is true and 0 otherwise.

Krause and Pinheiro (2007) combined the simulation idea with modeling and applied it to a post-hoc subgroup analysis of an Alzheimer study (Farlow et al., 2005). The dataset of interest comprised 679 patients that received placebo during the initial 26 weeks and switched to test treatment for the second 26 weeks, in an open label phase. It was observed that patients with a faster disease progression in the initial phase (rapidly progressing patients) showed a slower rate of disease progression in the open-label phase when compared to patients who had progressed more slowly in the initial phase (slow progressors). There is a risk that this observation could be due to regression to the mean.

The data for each patient comprises the cognitive score at baseline, after 26 weeks on placebo, and after 52 weeks with 26 weeks on active treatment. These are converted to change from baseline at week 26 and week 52, resulting in two observations per patient. Patients with a change from baseline at week 26 of 4 points or less (on a 70 point scale) were classified as slow progressors. Data for 517 patients were available at the end of the observation period. A regression analysis allowed to reject the hypothesis of equal progression after week 26 with a p-value of 0.0042. The adjusted p-value turned out to be 0.029, considerably less compelling than the observed one.

3.6 SIMPSON'S PARADOX

Simpson's paradox is an extreme condition of confounding in which an apparent association between two variables is reversed when the data are analyzed within each stratum of a confounding variable. The phenomenon was first described by Karl Pearson in 1899 and again some years later in 1903 by George Yule, but it was named after Edward Simpson who discussed it more thoroughly in 1951.

Consider the following situation: in a clinical study with 160 subjects, 80 receive a test drug (T) while the remaining 80 receive a control treatment (C). The objective of the study is to investigate whether the cure rate under T is higher than under C. The results of the study are shown in Table 3.3 suggesting an advantage of T over C.

Another person working on these data may wonder whether the results differ between male and female patients. After separating the data by gender the results shown in Table 3.4 are obtained. As a surprise, both men and women achieve a favorable result under C instead of T. How can T be more beneficial in the population as a whole and at the same time be harmful for each gender?

From a probabilistic point of view the paradox can be reformulated as follows:

$$\Pr[S|T] > \Pr[S|C] \qquad (3.3)$$

Table 3.3 Results of a fictitious study.

Treatment	Cured	Total	Cure rate
T	40	80	50%
C	32	80	40%

Table 3.4 Results of the fictitious study by gender.

Gender	Treatment	Cured	Total	Cure rate
Male	T	36	60	60%
	C	14	20	70%
Female	T	4	20	20%
	C	18	60	30%

$$\Pr[S|T, F] < \Pr[S|C, F] \qquad (3.4)$$

$$\Pr[S|T, M] < \Pr[S|C, M]. \qquad (3.5)$$

Here S denotes treatment success (cure), and F and M stand for female and male, respectively. Such a constellation is possible as long as the distribution of gender can depend on treatment. Otherwise the following result holds.

Theorem 3.1: *If* $\Pr[F|T] = \Pr[F|C] = \Pr[F]$, *(3.4) and (3.5) imply* $\Pr[S|T] < \Pr[S|C]$.

Proof: Note that $\Pr[M|T] = \Pr[M|C] = \Pr[M]$ since $\Pr[M|C] = 1 - \Pr[F|C]$ and $\Pr[M|T] = 1 - \Pr[F|T]$. Then the assertion follows from

$$\begin{aligned}\Pr[S|T] &= \Pr[S|T, F]\Pr[F|T] + \Pr[S|T, M]\Pr[M|T] \\ &= \Pr[S|T, F]\Pr[F] + \Pr[S|T, M]\Pr[M] \\ &< \Pr[S|C, F]\Pr[F] + \Pr[S|C, M]\Pr[M] \\ &= \Pr[S|C].\end{aligned}$$

In a randomized clinical trial with complete randomization, the assignment of treatment T

is independent of the other covariates, hence the assumption of the theorem is fulfilled. Consequently, at least in large randomized studies, the risk for Simpson's paradox to occur is small. However, in observational studies where treatment administration may be linked to a covariate like gender, the paradox is theoretically possible. In the artificial example above, a cure happened more often in men than in women regardless of the treatment taken, but more men took the treatment with lower chance of a cure (T) while more women took the treatment with higher chance of a cure (C). This imbalance is sufficient to reverse the treatment effect in the population as a whole.

3.7 POST-HOC ANALYSES

The pitfalls described so far constitute threats even for pre-specified subgroup analyses. The situation can only become worse for post-hoc analyses which aim to identify a part of the patient population with improved efficacy or benefit–risk profile compared to the entire study population after the study data are available.

The approach has the flavor of "betting on the horse when the race is over," an attempt entirely unacceptable in the betting business. Or, to quote Senn and Harrell (1997), "Hindsight is so much more precise than foresight and but for its unfortunate habit of arriving too late, it would surely be used for prediction all the time." As a consequence, it is natural to expect overstatements. The ISIS–2, BHAT and the Actimmune trials (see Chapter 1) are relevant examples in this context.

The question arises whether there is any reasonable approach to deal with post-hoc analyses to avoid fallacies. Lee and Rubin (2016) proposed a solution under the assumption that the subgroup selection mechanism is known. They exemplified it for the case of the Actimmune study. Their proposal bears some similarity to the regression to the mean corrected p-value of Krause and Pinheiro (2007). A simplified version goes like this:

1. Specify precisely the post-hoc subgrouping procedure, which leads to the selection of the subgroup with the smallest p-value.
2. Perform the post-hoc subgrouping procedure on the observed dataset to obtain the observed subgroup p-value p_{obs}.
3. Repeat the following steps for $m = 1, \ldots, M$:
   (a) Replace the treatment allocation in the original dataset with a randomly permuted assignment of treatment indicators.
   (b) Perform the post-hoc subgrouping procedure to obtain a p-value p_m.
4. The randomization based p-value is obtained from
$$p_{\text{adj}} = \frac{1}{M} \sum_{m=1}^{M} I(p_m \leq p_{\text{obs}})$$

where I denotes the indicator function with $I(A) = 1$ if A is true and 0 otherwise.

Applying this idea to the Actimmune data, the p-value of 0.004 as reported for the post-hoc subgroup analysis by InterMune increases to 0.04, still formally statistically significant. However, post-hoc subgrouping procedures incorporating secondary endpoints or additional covariates would likely have pushed the adjusted p-value to insignificance. This constitutes the crux of post-hoc analyses: it is rarely obvious which analyses have been performed before getting to the subgroup with a difference.

3.8 CONCLUDING REMARKS

The most severe issues in subgroup analyses likely occur in the situation when unplanned analyses are mainly driven by knowledge of the data of the study at hand. This does not mean that one should ignore the unforeseen results of an investigation because one has not thought about them in advance. Many groundbreaking discoveries have been made by chance (Ban, 2006; Hargrave-Thomas et al., 2012). However, the point is how these results are weighed and interpreted. One explanation that should always be considered is whether the observed effects can be explained by randomness or sampling and variation of the data.

In this chapter we discussed observations that call for a cause: a more extreme result, a reversal of observed effects, a change from baseline. Often, the explanation for these findings is statistical and not causal: small sample size, multiple analyses, imperfect correlation, and selection. Among the remedies are larger samples, control groups, randomization, and replication. It should not come as a surprise that many people with a skeptical view on subgroup analyses are statisticians.

There seems to be a psychological component as well. As Daniel Kahneman puts it: "Our predilection for causal thinking exposes us to serious mistakes in evaluating the randomness of truly random events... We are pattern seekers, believers in a coherent world, in which regularities... appear not by accident but as a result of mechanical causality or of someone's intention. We do not expect to see regularity produced by a random process, and when we detect what appears to be a rule, we quickly reject the idea that the process is truly random."(Kahneman, 2012)

4

Subgroup Analysis and Modeling

The sciences do not try to explain, they hardly even try to interpret, they mainly make models. By a model is meant a mathematical construct which, with the addition of certain verbal interpretations, describes observed phenomena. The justification of such a mathematical construct is solely and precisely that it is expected to work – that is, correctly to describe phenomena from a reasonably wide area. Furthermore, it must satisfy certain esthetic criteria – that is, in relation to how much it describes, it must be rather simple.

John von Neumann (1903–1957)

4.1 INTRODUCTION

In this chapter we discuss the relationship between exploratory subgroup analyses and statistical modeling in broad terms. As was pointed out earlier, subdividing the full dataset and analyzing the resulting subsets separately will lead to less accurate and potentially exaggerated effect estimators because of the smaller sample size. Relating covariates with the outcomes by means of a model enables sharing information across subgroups and to reduce variability. On the flip side, modeling requires additional assumptions that may be hard to verify or even rationalize at times.

In the following we consider mainly two types of models in some detail: hierarchical models and regression models. (Linear models are treated as regression models with binary or categorical covariates.)

Hierarchical models assume that the parameters describing the effect in the subgroups are drawn from a common distribution. This assumption allows defining, within a subgroup, estimators that are less variable than the original ones if the results in subgroups do not differ too much. As it turns out the hierarchical estimators are closer to the overall effect in the full dataset than the original estimators, a phenomenon that is called "shrinkage". The primary purpose of hierarchical models in subgroup analyses is therefore estimation of the effects in subgroups. This approach is pursued further in Chapter 5.

Regression models link the outcome of an intervention to some covariates. The strength of the impact of the covariates on the output is described by parameters in the model. If model parameters can be interpreted in regard to subgroups, estimation of the regression coefficients can be of primary interest. If the main purpose of modeling is to predict the outcome of future subjects, minimizing the prediction error is more important than optimizing the estimators of coefficients.

Regression models lend themselves to variable selection to retain only those variables in the model that affect the outcome. Since variables relate to subgroups, variable selection corresponds to identifying the most relevant subgroups.

4.2 MODELING AND PREDICTION

Following Breiman (2001), the basic paradigm is that data are generated by a black box ("nature") in which independent variables $\mathbf{X}$ go in one side and a response Y comes out the other. The potential goals of statistical analyses are:

1. To extract information about how the response variables are associated to the input variables.
2. To predict the responses of future input variables.

The first approach is called *data modeling*, the second *prediction*. A data model relates outcome to input variables, model parameters, and additional random elements ("noise"). A predictor can also be defined in terms of a regression model or more generally in terms of decision trees, neural nets, etc.

Model validation can principally be achieved by assessing goodness-of-fit or prediction accuracy. One issue with goodness-of-fit tests is their low power, i.e. the deviations of the model and the unknown association of the data have to be large to be detected (Bickel et al., 2006). On the other hand, when the sample size is large, irrelevant deviations may become significant. The other problem is the dichotomy of the method: a model either fits or does not fit.

A fit gets generally better for more complex rather than simple models. To reflect this, goodness-of-fit measures have been developed that account for model complexity. Examples are the Akaike information criterion (AIC) (Akaike, 1973) or the Bayesian information criterion (BIC) (Schwartz, 1979). They penalize the apparent model fit as expressed by means of the model likelihood ℓ for model complexity as follows:

$$\text{AIC} = -2 \log \ell(\hat{\theta}) + 2q \qquad (4.1)$$

$$\text{BIC} = -2 \log \ell(\hat{\theta}) + q \log(M). \qquad (4.2)$$

Here q denotes the number of parameters in the model and M the number of subjects for linear models, or the number of events for survival data or number of less frequent outcome for binary data (Heinze et al., 2018). Smaller values indicate a better fit. Since for any realistic sample size the penalty factor for the BIC is larger than that of the

AIC, the BIC tends to prefer less complex models. Hence applying different criteria can result in different optimal models for the same data. However, even the same criterion can suggest a similar goodness-of-fit for rather different models.

Following Breiman (2001), a more obvious way to check how well a model emulates the black box is this:

1. Put a case **X** down the black box getting an output Y.
2. Put the same case down the model getting an output Y'.
3. The closeness of Y and Y' is a measure of how good the prediction is.

However, as with goodness-of-fit, if the model is too complex, it may overfit the data and give an over-optimistic impression of precision. Luckily, there are ways to remove this type of bias by cross-validation (Stone, 1974) and bootstrap methods (Efron, 1983; Efron and Tibshirani, 1997). We get back to the concept of prediction in Chapter 8.

Another aspect of the trade-off between accuracy and complexity is interpretability of results. A highly accurate model containing a lot of variables may still be perceived as a black box that provides little help to understanding why a specific prediction is made. Also for practical reasons a predictor involving only a few variables is preferable, particularly if assessments are expensive or complicated.

4.3 SUBGROUPS AND HIERARCHICAL MODELS

4.3.1 Stein's Discovery

For centuries the following result going back to Gauss (1777–1855) was undisputed:

Theorem 4.1: *For $n = 1, \ldots, N$, let Y_n be independently normally distributed random variables with means μ_n and variance 1. Then Y_n is the minimum variance unbiased estimator of μ_n.*

However, when one is prepared to give in on unbiasedness, Stein (1956) showed that one can do better in terms of variance:

Theorem 4.2: *Under the conditions of Theorem 4.1 let*

$$\hat{\mu}_n = \left(1 - \frac{b}{a + \sum_{n=1}^{N} Y_n^2}\right) Y_n$$

with $a, b > 0$. Then, for $N \geq 3$, a and b can be chosen such that

$$\sum_{n=1}^{N} E[(\hat{\mu}_n - \mu_n)^2] < N = \sum_{n=1}^{N} E[(Y_n - \mu_n)^2]$$

i.e. that the squared error loss of $(\hat{\mu}_1, \ldots, \hat{\mu}_N)$ is smaller than that of $(Y_1, \ldots, Y_N)$.

Stein's result shows primarily the existence of better, i.e. less variable estimators, than the maximum likelihood estimator if more than two groups of data are concerned. The trick is to appropriately use the sum of squares of *all* data for the estimation of an *individual* parameter. Unfortunately the theorem does not provide an explicit formula for such an estimator. Furthermore the result does not imply $E[(\hat{\mu}_n - \mu_n)^2] < E[(Y_n - \mu_n)^2]$ individually for all n.

A closed form estimator was provided some years later by James and Stein (1961) where the authors showed that the squared error loss of

$$\hat{\mu}_n = \left(1 - \frac{N-2}{\sum_{n=1}^{N} Y_n^2}\right) Y_n$$

is smaller than N for $N \geq 3$. However, the James–Stein estimator is still not the one with the smallest possible variance.

Notably, the authors obtained their results without assuming a hierarchical model nor referring to Bayesian reasoning. In fact the results have been derived by entirely frequentist thinking. Nevertheless they paved the way to what was then called empirical Bayes estimation.

4.3.2 The Normal–Normal Hierarchical Model

We recall here the simplest hierarchical model suitable for subgroup analysis. Denote by θ_k the effects of an intervention in subset S_k of the total population, $k = 1, \ldots, K$. Let Z_k be an unbiased estimate of θ_k with

$$Z_k | \theta_k, \sigma_k^2 \sim N(\theta_k, \sigma_k^2)$$

for known variances σ_k^2.

This assumption is fairly widely applicable since it holds at least asymptotically for maximum likelihood estimators. For example, in a survival study comparing a new intervention with a control, θ_k can be defined as the log hazard ratio between the two treatments in S_k. Let d_k be the total number of events in subgroup S_k. Under a 1:1 randomization among treatments $\sigma_k^2 = d_k/4$ (Schoenfeld, 1983). For binary data the log odds ratio is a parameter of choice. Also, in one of the examples considered later, standard normal z statistics occur such that $\sigma_k = 1$ for all units. We further assume that the θ_k are from a normal distribution with

$$\theta_k | \eta, \tau^2 \sim N(\eta, \tau^2). \qquad (4.3)$$

Note that (4.3) does not require independence of θ_k but only exchangeability, i.e. that any vector obtained by permuting the elements of $(\theta_1, \ldots, \theta_K)$ has the same distribution as the original vector. This is the case if the correlation of any pairs (θ_k, θ_l) is identical.

The marginal distribution of Z_k is then given by

$$Z_k \sim N(\eta, \sigma_k^2 + \tau^2)$$

Subgroups and Hierarchical Models

and the posterior distribution of θ_k is normal with mean

$$\theta_k(z) = E[\theta_k|Z_k = z] = \omega_k z + (1 - \omega_k)\eta \quad (4.4)$$

and variance

$$\sigma_k^2(z) = V[\theta_k|Z_k = z] = \omega_k \sigma_k^2 \quad (4.5)$$

with weights

$$0 \le \omega_k = \frac{\tau^2}{\sigma_k^2 + \tau^2} \le 1. \quad (4.6)$$

The posterior mean $\theta_k(z)$ in (4.4) is a convex combination of the estimator Z_k for subgroup S_k and the parameter η that shrinks an estimator of θ_k towards the overall mean. At the same time, it also reduces the posterior variance (4.5) of all subgroup estimators.

If τ^2 is very large, i.e. the effects differ much among subgroups, $\omega_k \approx 1$ and $\theta_k(z)$ is just derived from data in S_k. This is reasonable since the data from other subgroups would not provide valuable information to help improving the estimator for θ_k.

If τ^2 is close to zero, i.e. the subgroup effects θ_k are practically identical, $\omega_k \approx 0$, and the posterior expectations of all θ_k are identical to η independently of the observed estimators Z_k. In this case the best estimator of a subgroup effect is the overall effect.

Eventually, if the group effect estimators are very precise, i.e. if $\sigma_k^2 \approx 0$, it follows that $\omega_k \approx 1$ and there is no gain by shifting estimators towards η. In any case it should be noted that because of (4.6)

$$\sigma_k^2(z) \leq \min\{\sigma_k^2, \tau^2\}.$$

Therefore the posterior variance of *every* θ_k is smaller than the variance of Z_k and smaller than the between group variance τ^2. Thus hierarchical modeling allows for effect estimates with smaller variances than the original per group estimates in the spirit of Stein's findings.

4.4 SUBGROUPS AND REGRESSION MODELS

4.4.1 Subgroups Defined in Terms of Variables

Assume that each of $n = 1, \ldots, N$ individuals in a study can be characterized by a set of K covariates $\mathbf{X}_n = (X_{1n}, \ldots, X_{Kn})$. The outcome in individual n under treatment $T_n \in \{0, 1\}$ is denoted by Y_n. If not otherwise stated, T_n is supposed to be independent of the covariates $\mathbf{X}_n$, which is the case in randomized studies. $\mathcal{L} = \{(Y_n, \mathbf{X}_n, T_n), n = 1, \ldots, N\}$ is called a *learning dataset*.

If X_{kn} are binary or categorical, subgroups can be defined in terms of covariates, for example

$$S_k^+ = \{n; X_{nk} = 1\}, \quad S_k^- = \{n; X_{nk} = 0\} \quad (4.7)$$

for univariate subgroups. By linking subgroups and covariates in such a way, the task to identify subgroups of patients that benefit more from treatment than others is equivalent to selecting relevant covariates.

A relatively simple but fairly flexible approach is to fit some function of the expectation of Y_n by a linear predictor in terms of the covariates, a generalized linear model (GLIM) (Diggle et al., 2002; Molenberghs and Verbeke, 2005):

$$h(E[Y|\mathbf{x}, t]) = \eta(\mathbf{x}, t)$$
$$= \alpha + \beta t + \sum_{k=1}^{K} \gamma_k x_k + t \sum_{k=1}^{K} \delta_k x_k. \quad (4.8)$$

For normally distributed Y, the link function h is the identity. For binary outcome data, typical link functions are the logit function $h(p) = p/(1-p)$ or the probit function $h(p) = \Phi^{-1}(p)$ where $p = E[Y]$ and Φ denotes the cdf of a standard normal variable. Parameters in GLIMs can be estimated by a (restricted) maximum likelihood estimation. For survival data, one could fit a proportional hazards model (Cox, 1972):

$$\lambda(y; \mathbf{x}, t) = \lambda_0(y) \exp\{\eta(\mathbf{x}, t)\}. \quad (4.9)$$

Parameter estimates can be obtained from maximizing a partial likelihood (Cox, 1975).

To understand the meaning of the coefficients in the linear predictor let $\mathbf{x}_k(i) =$

$(x_1, \ldots, x_{k-1}, i, x_{k+1}, \ldots, x_K)$. Then

$$\eta(\mathbf{x}_k(1), 0) - \eta(\mathbf{x}_k(0), 0) = \gamma_k \qquad (4.10)$$

i.e. γ_k equals the treatment effect of control treatment in S_k^+ relative to S_k^- given that all other covariates are identical. γ_k is called a *prognostic effect*. For the test treatment it follows that

$$\eta(\mathbf{x}_k(1), 1) - \eta(\mathbf{x}_k(0), 1) = \gamma_k + \delta_k. \qquad (4.11)$$

Hence δ_k is the difference of (4.11) and (4.10) what can be rewritten as

$$\delta_k = \eta(\mathbf{x}_k(1), 1) - \eta(\mathbf{x}_k(1), 0) \\ - [\eta(\mathbf{x}_k(0), 1) - \eta(\mathbf{x}_k(0), 0)]$$

i.e. the difference between the effect differences of test versus control in S_k^+ and S_k^-, respectively. δ_k is called a *predictive effect*. If $\delta_k = 0$, the difference in test and control is identical on either subset and thus there is no reason for a subset specific preference of test over control. If $\delta_k \neq 0$, the difference between test treatment and control differs across subgroups. Therefore the parameters δ_k (the treatment by subgroup interactions) are of major importance for subgroup analysis. However, $\delta_k \neq 0$ could still mean that test is better (or worse) than control in the entire patient population, but remarkably better (or worse) in a subset. This interaction is called *quantitative*. If the test is better

Subgroups and Regression Models

than the control in one subset but worse than control in the other, i.e. if

$$\eta(\mathbf{x}_k(1), 1) - \eta(\mathbf{x}_k(1), 0) < 0$$
$$< \eta(\mathbf{x}_k(0), 1) - \eta(\mathbf{x}_k(0), 0) \qquad (4.12)$$

or with inequalities reversed, the interaction is called *qualitative* interaction. In such a situation the correct treatment assignment is crucial. Now

$$\eta(\mathbf{x}_k(1), 1) - \eta(\mathbf{x}_k(1), 0) = \beta + \delta_k + \sum_{l \neq k} \delta_l x_l$$

$$\eta(\mathbf{x}_k(0), 1) - \eta(\mathbf{x}_k(0), 0) = \beta + \sum_{l \neq k} \delta_l x_l.$$

Hence (4.12) is equivalent to

$$\delta_k < -\beta - \sum_{l \neq k} \delta_l x_l < 0$$

which is a stronger requirement than the condition $\delta_k < 0$. Figures 4.1–4.3 visualize the different types of interaction. In all cases, it is assumed that all but the kth covariates are identical in both subsets.

4.4.2 The Predicted Individual Treatment Effect

Another way to define subgroups utilizes the predicted individual treatment effect (PITE). For covariates $\mathbf{x}$ and treatment t let $Y(\mathbf{x}, t)$ be the potential outcome of a subject with covariates $\mathbf{x}$

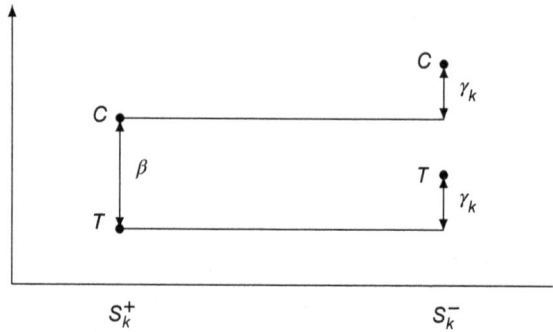

Figure 4.1 No treatment by subgroup interaction: constant difference β between T and C across subgroups, but potentially different effects of T and C across subgroups as reflected by γ_k.

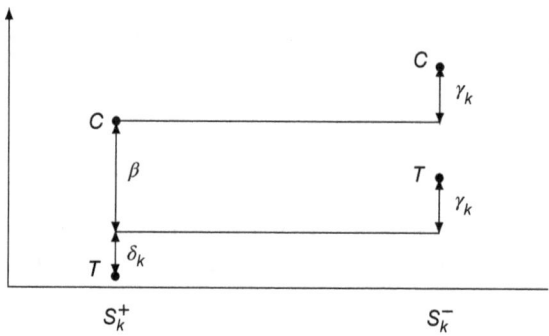

Figure 4.2 Example of quantitative treatment by subgroup interaction: difference between T and C varies across subgroups as reflected by δ_k on top of the common difference γ_k, but T is always superior to C.

receiving treatment t. Then the PITE is defined by (Cai et al., 2011; Chen et al., 2017; Lamont et al., 2018)

$$D(\mathbf{x}) = E[Y(\mathbf{x}, 1)] - E[Y(\mathbf{x}, 0)].$$

Subgroups and Regression Models

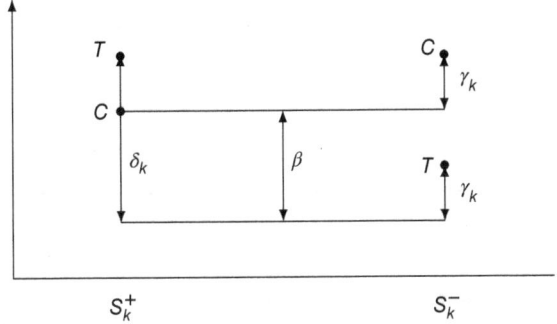

Figure 4.3 Example of qualitative treatment by subgroup interaction: difference between T and C varies across subgroups as reflected by $\delta_k \geq \beta > 0$ on top of the common difference γ_k, but T is superior to C on S_k^- and inferior on S_k^+.

Given the appropriate PITE one can set a threshold c to define a subset

$$S(c) = \{\mathbf{x}; D(\mathbf{x}) \leq c\}. \qquad (4.13)$$

The threshold c should reflect a clinically relevant effect to be defined by clinicians, regulators, or policy makers.

With this approach, the covariate space is always split into two parts regardless of the number of covariates with the test treatment being remarkably better than the control in the subset defined by (4.13) and not so much better or even worse in the complementary subset. The subsets obtained directly from covariates and those obtained via the PITE are visualized in Figures 4.4 and 4.5.

82 Subgroup Analysis and Modeling

	$X_1 = 0, X_2 = 0$	$X_1 = 1, X_2 = 0$
0		
1	$X_1 = 0, X_2 = 1$	$X_1 = 1, X_2 = 1$

$$0 \qquad\qquad 1$$

	$X_1 < x_1, X_2 < x_2$	$X_1 \geq x_1, X_2 < x_2$
x_2		
	$X_1 < x_1, X_2 \geq x_2$	$X_1 \geq x_1, X_2 \geq x_2$

$$x_1$$

Figure 4.4 Subgroups defined by two binary (upper diagram) or two numerical covariates X_1 and X_2 with corresponding thresholds x_1 and x_2 (lower diagram).

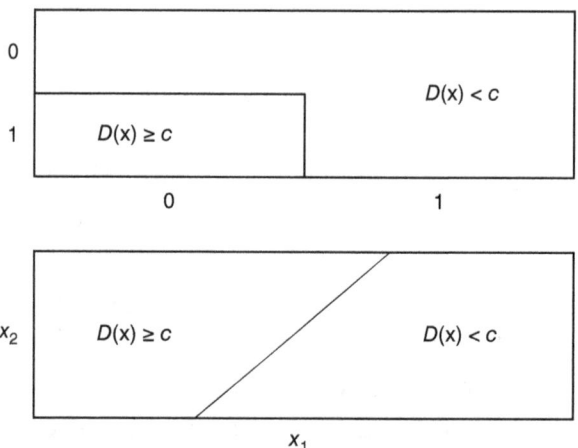

Figure 4.5 Subgroups defined by the individual treatment effect in the case of two binary (upper diagram) or two numerical covariates (lower diagram). In either case only two subgroups are obtained.

The definition of a PITE can be generalized to binary or count data by

$$D(\mathbf{x}) = h\{E[Y(\mathbf{x}, 1)]\} - h\{E[Y(\mathbf{x}, 0)]\} \quad (4.14)$$

for some link function h (see Diggle et al. (2002), Molenberghs and Verbeke (2005)) or by

$$D(\mathbf{x}) = \log\{\lambda(y; \mathbf{x}, 1)\} - \log\{\lambda(y; \mathbf{x}, 0)\}$$

for survival data. In each case, one obtains for linear predictors

$$D(\mathbf{x}) = \eta(\mathbf{x}, 1) - \eta(\mathbf{x}, 0) = \beta + \sum_{k=1}^{K} \delta_k x_k$$

i.e. the PITE depends only on the overall treatment effect β and the treatment by covariate interaction effects δ_k.

One can further characterize the shape of the subsets $S(c)$ for linear predictors. For continuous covariates $\mathbf{X} \in R^K$, $S(c)$ is separated from its complement by a the $(K-1)$-dimensional hyperplane $H(c) = \{\mathbf{x}; D(\mathbf{x}) = c\}$. For $K=1$ one obtains $S(c) = \{x; \beta + \delta x \geq c\}$, leading to a dichotomization of X at $(c-\beta)/\delta$. For $K=2$, $S(c) = \{(x_1, x_2); \beta + \delta_1 x_1 + \delta_2 x_2 \geq c\}$ consists of all points above a straight line through $((c-\beta)/\delta_1, 0)$ and $(0, (c-\beta)/\delta_2)$.

4.4.3 Comparison of the Two Options

The two options of defining subgroups have advantages and disadvantages. The marginal thresholds used under the first approach are easy to interpret and the subgroups are defined in a straightforward manner based on the original data. However, the approach can generate very large numbers of subsets even for moderate numbers of covariates.

Defining subgroups via covariates is straightforward for binary covariates but requires categorization for continuous covariates. It is known that dichotomizing a continuous confounder in ordinary regression can result in biased estimation (Cumsille et al., 2000). As shown in Austin and Brunner (2004) an inflation of the type I error rate occurs when testing a continuous factor after adjusting for a correlated continuous confounding variable that has been divided into categories. Interestingly this increase occurs with increasing sample size, increasing correlation between the factor of interest and the confounder with a decrease in the number of categories into which the confounder is divided. As a result, a factor in the model may be identified as relevant and utilized to define subgroups just because a confounder has been categorized. Eventually, there is the idea to define "optimal" cutpoints to obtain categories that maximize the impact of a covariate; however this kind of optimality will not hold beyond the sample analyzed (Royston et al., 2006). Therefore, whenever possible, categories should be pre-defined based on experience.

If interactions rather than direct effects in subgroups are to be considered, modeling may be required. Basing decisions on tests for differences within groups or interactions emphasizes statistical significance rather than relevance.

The approach using the PITE defines subgroups in terms of relevant expected outcomes rather than covariate related thresholds. It divides the covariance space in two subsets regardless of the number of covariates. However it requires modeling and may lead to rather unintuitive relationships between effects and covariates, in particular when the number of covariates is large.

4.5 VARIABLE SELECTION IN REGRESSION

Whenever data are to be described by a regression model there is concern about the model type (e.g., linear versus non-linear) or the covariates to be included in the model. There are good reasons to prefer models with a small number of covariates, so-called *sparse* models. From a statistical point of view, non-predictive covariates are adding mainly noise but no signal and should therefore not be considered in the first place. Second, a relationship between a small number of covariates and an outcome of interest is just easier to interpret.

On the other hand, forgetting relevant variables in a statistical model can also cause issues. When the assumptions of linear regression apply, adjustment of covariates that are associated with the response variable is not required to obtain a valid (i.e. consistent and/or unbiased) estimate of a treatment effect. However, adjustment is desirable as it will improve the precision of the effect estimate, as long as these covariates are not correlated ("confounded"). In logistic regression models or proportional hazards models, this may even happen for uncorrelated variables (Robinson and Jewell, 1991). Even worse, omitting relevant covariates in non-linear regression models results in biased effects estimators (Gail et al., 1984; Hauck et al., 1998). This holds also for survival data (Schmoor and Schumacher, 1997).

4.5.1 Classical Variable Selection

Variable selection requires selection criteria and a selection algorithm that defines how the criteria are to be applied (Heinze et al., 2018). The most prominent algorithms are backward elimination or forward selection or a combination of them. Backward elimination starts with a full model, i.e. a model including all candidate variables, and eliminates variables if an elimination criterion is fulfilled. In contrast, forward selection starts with a null model containing only the intercept and adds variables according to specified selection criteria. In stepwise selection a selection step and an elimination step alternate. The best subset selection tries to identify the most appropriate model out of 2^K possible models.

There are different kinds of criteria for inclusion or removal of covariates. One option is tests for the hypotheses $H_K : \delta_k = 0$. A variable is included into the model if the corresponding P-value is below some threshold $0 < \alpha_S < 1$ or removed from the model if it is above $0 < \alpha_R < 1$. Another option is to use information criteria like the Akaike information criterion (AIC) (Akaike, 1973) or the Bayesian information criterion (BIC) (Schwartz, 1979) already introduced earlier. Variables are included into the model as long as they reduce the AIC or the BIC.

4.5.2 Regularized Estimators

Instead of using a selection criterion in a sequential variable selection procedure one can build penalization into the parameter estimation process. A well known method in this regard is the LASSO (least absolute shrinkage and selection operator) first introduced in the context of least squares estimation in linear models (Tibshirani, 1996) and later generalized to maximum likelihood estimation (Tibshirani, 1997). Given observations $(y_n, \mathbf{x}_n)$, the objective of the LASSO is to

$$\text{minimize } \frac{1}{N} \sum_{n=1}^{N} (y_n - \beta_0 - \mathbf{x}_n^t \beta)^2$$

$$\text{subject to } \sum_{k=1}^{K} |\beta_k| \leq r$$

where $r > 0$ is the regularization parameter. Regularization in this way results in parameter estimates of zero for small parameters and thus in model selection. At the same time large estimates are shrunken towards zero. For this process to work appropriately the covariates should be standardized such that all estimates are on the same scale. The regularization parameter can be selected using cross-validation.

Defining valid confidence intervals for model parameters from LASSO fits is not trivial and was an open problem for a while until the publication of (Hastie et al., 2015) and still has open questions (see for example Kivaranovic and Leeb (2018)). We will follow up this discussion in Chapter 7.

4.5.3 Variable Selection and Confounding

In a setting with several baseline covariates, the interpretation of a regression coefficient is that of the expected change in outcome if one variable X_k changes by one unit and all other variables are held constant. If X_k is correlated with the other covariates, the size and therefore the interpretation of the corresponding regression coefficient changes under variable selection.

An illustrative example of this phenomenon is presented in Heinze et al. (2018). They considered a model explaining the relationship between the percentage of body fat and weight, height, and abdomen circumference, three obviously correlated covariates. Table 4.1 shows regression coefficients from four different models.

Table 4.1 Estimates and standard errors of regression coefficients from four different models for the body fat data

Model	Weight (kg)	Height (cm)	Abdomen (cm)	R^2
1	0.420 (0.034)			0.381
2	0.582 (0.034)	−0.586 (0.062)		0.543
3	−0.292 (0.047)		0.979 (0.056)	0.722
4	−0.215 (0.068)	−0.096 (0.062)	0.910 (0.071)	0.723

Note that the intercept has been dropped from the table. R^2 denotes the adjusted coefficient of determination.

One realizes that the coefficient of weight changes considerably in magnitude and even in sign if different covariates are entered in the model. The factor height can be deemed important or irrelevant depending on whether abdomen circumference was adjusted for or not.

4.6 CONCLUDING REMARKS

Variable selection will hardly provide the best of all possible models, but the most appropriate within a class of candidate models defined by the model type and the input variables. An important variable that has been forgotten at the outset will not be identified during a model selection process. At best the incomplete model will result in a fit with inefficient parameter estimates, otherwise it may produce biased estimates. May be this observation encourages to start with more complex models and let model selection procedures do the job to weed out variables that do not add value. However, the model selection criterion and the algorithm chosen will to some extend decide on what is important.

The impact of missing important covariates differs between model types. Linear models are robust in the sense that the variability of estimators increases when variables are omitted but the means are sill estimated correctly. Parameter estimates in nonlinear models like GLIMs or the proportional hazard models are getting severely biased in these circumstances.

As a consequence it is extremely important to check the results of modeling for plausibility and meaningfulness. Following Wallach et al. (2017), corroboration of subgroup analyses is hardly performed and the results are not encouraging in cases where it was done.

5

Hierarchical Models in Subgroup Analysis

Surely there is no one among us who believes that a sample of data from a normal distribution has ever existed. One hopes that the models belief is also universally held to be true. Any analyst who has fitted a straight line through some data has either done so knowing that it was only a reasonable approximation to the true relationship or has remembered the dire text-book warnings of extrapolation beyond the range of the data. (Nester, 1996).

Marks R. Nester, An Applied Statisticians Creed

5.1 INTRODUCTION

The methods to be presented in this chapter are most suited to estimate the effects in subgroups by utilizing information from other subgroups where possible. This information sharing can compensate for the lower precision of effect estimators in subgroups caused by the smaller number of subjects as compared to the entire study. Hierarchical models provide the framework for such an effort but rely on additional distributional assumptions.

As originally shown in Stein (1956), estimating a number of effects individually (e.g., by maximum likelihood or least squares) is not optimal in the sense of squared error loss. This result triggered the branch of empirical Bayes (EB) estimation (Robbins, 1956, Morris, 1983, Efron and Morris, 1973,1975; Carlin and Louis, 2000, Greenland, 2000).

Empirical Bayes estimation has been applied in the medical setting to meta analysis (DerSimonian and Laird, 1986), estimation of efficacy in subgroups (Davis and Leffingwell, 1990), to the analysis of spontaneous reporting data of adverse reactions of approved drugs (DuMouchel, 1999), and analysis of adverse events in clinical trials (Rosenkranz, 2010). The role of the EB methodology in medical research has been recently reviewed in a broader context (van Houwelingen, 2014). Alternative approaches to subgroup analyses like Bayesian hierarchical models have been proposed for subgroup identification and detection of interactions (Bayman et al., 2010, Berger et al., 2014, Jones et al., 2011, Varadhan and Wang, 2016).

The common denominator of these examples is the intention to increase the precision of the estimators of (sub)group effects where sample sizes are smaller than in the entire study by borrowing information across groups. The extent to which this is possible is determined by the between group variability. Another aspect mainly apparent in meta analyses is the quest for an overall treatment effect from several studies.

Most of the earlier applications of hierarchical models to stratified analyses rely on the exchangeability of all subgroup effects. This implies that their estimators are identically distributed. Generalizations have been considered as well, among them a mixture of two gamma distributions (DuMouchel, 1999) or a normal mixture prior (Rosenkranz, 2010). The interpretations of mixture priors are diverse. The pragmatic argument goes that more components allow for more flexibility without attributing the components to some real world features of the data (DuMouchel, 1999). Second, considering different groups of exchangeable and non-exchangeable variables may provide a more appropriate description of the data (Neuenschwander et al., 2015). Third, a wide range of prior distributions can be approximated by a weighted average of conjugate priors (Dalal and Hall, 1983, Schmidli et al., 2014). In the case where disjoint clusters of exchangeable group effects exist the notion of an overall effect may become less meaningful. A disadvantage of a more complex model is obviously the higher number of parameters to be estimated and a risk of over-fitting. Therefore it would be good to find criteria that help in determining the most appropriate degree of model complexity in a specific situation.

5.2 A GENERAL HIERARCHICAL MODEL

5.2.1 Robbins' Theorem and Tweedie's Formula

In Section 4.3 we introduced the simplest hierarchical model suitable for subgroup analysis: denote by θ_k the effects of an intervention in subset S_k, $k = 1, \ldots, K$, and let Z_k be an unbiased estimate of θ_k with

$$Z_k | \theta_k, \sigma_k^2 \sim N(\theta_k, \sigma_k^2)$$

for known variances σ_k^2. We further assumed that the θ_k are from a normal distribution with

$$\theta_k | \eta, \tau^2 \sim N(\eta, \tau^2).$$

In this section we relax the conditions on the prior of the treatment effects θ_k, but stick to the assumption $Z_k \sim N(\theta_k, \sigma_k^2)$ since it covers maximum likelihood effect estimators, at least asymptotically. First we state a general result on the posterior expectations and variances of empirical Bayes estimators, originally presented in Robbins (1956):

Theorem 5.1: *Let $\theta \sim g(\cdot)$ an arbitrary prior and $Z|\theta \sim N(\theta, \sigma^2)$ with σ known. Let $f(z)$ denote the marginal distribution of Z, i.e.*

$$f(z) = \frac{1}{\sigma} \int \phi\left(\frac{z-\theta}{\sigma}\right) g(\theta) d\theta. \qquad (5.1)$$

Then

$$\theta(z) = E[\theta|Z=z] = z + \sigma^2 \frac{d \log f(z)}{dz} \qquad (5.2)$$

$$\sigma^2(z) = V[\theta|Z=z] = \sigma^2 \left[1 + \sigma^2 \frac{d^2 \log f(z)}{dz^2}\right]. \qquad (5.3)$$

A proof can be found in Robbins (1956) or Efron (2011). Equation (5.2) was first established in Tweedie (1947) and is therefore called Tweedie's formula. Both equations above are helpful in calculating or estimating the posterior expectation or variance of θ_k from the marginal distribution of Z_k. In particular when $\sigma_k = \sigma$ for all k, Z_k is identically distributed and the parameters thereof can be estimated from the empirical distribution of $(Z_1, \ldots, Z_K)$ without reference to the prior.

We apply the theorem to obtain the posterior mean and variance for the normal hierarchical model. Since the marginal probability density function of Z_k for the single component prior is given by

$$f_k(z) = c \exp\left\{-\frac{(z-\eta)^2}{2(\sigma_k^2 + \tau^2)}\right\}$$

one obtains with $c' = \log(c)$

$$\log f_k(z) = c' - \frac{(z-\eta)^2}{2(\sigma_k^2 + \tau^2)}$$

and

$$\frac{d\log f_k(z)}{dz} = -\frac{z-\eta}{\sigma_k^2 + \tau^2},$$

$$\frac{d^2\log f_k(z)}{dz^2} = -\frac{1}{\sigma_k^2 + \tau^2} < 0$$

Equations (4.4) and (4.5) of the previous chapter can now be easily obtained:

$$E[\theta_k|Z_k = z] = z - (z-\eta)\frac{\sigma_k^2}{\sigma_k^2 + \tau^2}$$

$$= \omega_k z + (1 - \omega_k)\eta$$

$$V[\theta_k|Z_k = z] = \sigma_k^2\left[1 + \sigma_k^2\left(-\frac{1}{\sigma_k^2 + \tau^2}\right)\right] = \omega_k \sigma_k^2.$$

In the remaining part of this and in the next section we will derive results for EB estimates from Theorem 5.1 above.

A General Hierarchical Model

Corollary 5.1: *Under the conditions of Theorem 5.1 it follows:*

1. *$\theta(z)$ is non-decreasing in z.*
2. *$V[\theta|Z = z] \leq \sigma^2$ if the marginal distribution $f(z)$ (5.1) is log concave.*

Proof: The first assertion follows from (5.2), (5.3) and

$$\frac{d\theta(z)}{dz} = 1 + \sigma^2 \frac{d^2 \log f(z)}{dz^2} = \frac{\sigma^2(z)}{\sigma^2} \geq 0$$

the second is immediate from (5.3).

It was shown above that $f(z)$ is log concave for the model with a normal prior. However this condition is not generally fulfilled for general priors like the mixture priors considered in the next section. This implies that the uniform variance reduction does not hold in general as will become obvious as a consequence of Corollary 5.2 and from the analysis of a dataset in Section 5.4.3.

5.2.2 Mixture Priors

In the following we consider mixtures of a point mass at 0 and normal distributions like

$$g(\theta) = \pi_0 \delta_0(\theta) + \sum_{j=1}^{J} \frac{\pi_j}{\tau_j} \phi\left(\frac{\theta - \eta_j}{\tau_j}\right) \qquad (5.4)$$

with $0 < \pi_j < 1$, $\sum_{j=0}^{J} \pi_j = 1$. The point mass is defined by $\delta_0(\Theta) = 1$ if $0 \in \Theta$ and zero if $0 \notin \Theta$ for any subset Θ of the parameter space. The first term in (5.4) accounts for the units that show no effect at all, the "null cases", and π_0 is the proportion of these units. Since

$$\eta_0 = \int \theta \delta_0(\theta) d\theta = 0, \quad \tau_0^2 = \int \theta^2 \delta_0(\theta) d\theta = 0$$

one obtains for the expectation of θ_k

$$\eta_J = E[\theta_k | \pi, \eta] = \sum_{j=1}^{J} \pi_j \eta_j \qquad (5.5)$$

and its variance

$$\tau_J^2 = V[\theta_k | \pi, \eta, \tau^2] = \sum_{j=0}^{J} \pi_j [\tau_j^2 + (\eta_j - \eta_J)^2]$$

$$= \pi_0 \eta_J^2 + \sum_{j=1}^{J} \pi_j [\tau_j^2 + (\eta_j - \eta_J)^2]. \qquad (5.6)$$

We further assume that there is an estimator Z_k of θ_k with

$$Z_k | \theta_k, \sigma_k \sim N(\theta_k, \sigma_k^2).$$

The marginal distribution of Z_k is then given by

$$Z_k \sim \pi_0 N(0, \sigma_k) + \sum_{j=1}^{J} \pi_j N(\eta_j, \sigma_i^2 + \tau_j^2) \qquad (5.7)$$

with

$$E[Z_k] = \eta_J, \quad V[Z_k] = \sigma_k^2 + \tau_J^2.$$

A General Hierarchical Model

Let

$$\phi_{kj}(z) = \frac{1}{(\sigma_k^2 + \tau_j^2)^{1/2}} \phi \left\{ \frac{z - \eta_j}{(\sigma_k^2 + \tau_j^2)^{1/2}} \right\}$$

and

$$f_k(z) = \sum_{j=0}^{J} \pi_j \phi_{kj}(z)$$

then $Q_{kj}(z)$, the posterior probability that θ_k is from the jth component of the mixture given $Z_k = z$, can be written as

$$Q_{kj}(z) = \frac{\pi_j \phi_{kj}(z)}{f_k(z)}. \qquad (5.8)$$

Then the following result holds:

Corollary 5.2: *For a hierarchical model with a mixture prior (5.4) the posterior mean and variance of θ_i are given by*

$$\theta_k(z) = \sum_{j=1}^{J} Q_{kj}(z)[\omega_{kj} z + (1 - \omega_{kj})\eta_j] \qquad (5.9)$$

and

$$\sigma_k^2(z) = \sum_{j=0}^{J} Q_{kj}(z)[\omega_{kj} z + (1 - \omega_{kj})\eta_j - \theta_k(z)]^2$$

$$+ \sigma_k^2 \sum_{j=0}^{J} Q_{kj}(z)\omega_{kj} \qquad (5.10)$$

with weights

$$\omega_{kj} = \frac{\tau_j^2}{\sigma_k^2 + \tau_j^2}. \quad (5.11)$$

For a proof see Rosenkranz (2018). It is obvious that the second term in (5.10) is always less than or equal to σ_k^2. However, the first term is always non-negative such that constellations of parameters are possible with $\sigma_k^2(z) > \sigma_k^2$ for some z.

5.2.3 The False Discovery Rate

The posterior probability that θ_k belongs to the "null" cases for $Z_k = z$ is the local false discovery rate given $Z_k = z$ (Efron, 2007),

$$\text{fdr}_k(z) = \Pr[\text{null}|Z_k = z] = Q_{k0}(z) = \frac{\pi_0 \phi_{k0}(z)}{f_k(z)}.$$

Let Φ_{k0} and F_k be the cumulative distribution functions corresponding to ϕ_{k0} and f_k, then the right sided tail area Fdr given $Z_k = z$ is

$$\text{Fdr}_k(z) = \Pr[\text{null}|Z_k \geq z] = \frac{\pi_0[1 - \Phi_{k0}(z)]}{1 - F_k(z)}. \quad (5.12)$$

The false discovery rate quantifies the proportion of subsets with an outcome $Z_k \geq z$ belonging to the null component. It correctly reflects the risk of a false positive decision given the data. This distinguishes the Fdr from the *p*-value, which quantifies the probability of the event $Z_k \geq z$ under the assumption $\theta_k = 0$. In fact, $1 - \Phi_{k0}(z)$ could be interpreted as the *p*-value of the hypothesis

$H_k : \theta_k = 0$. Equation (5.12) shows that the Fdr can be much larger than the p-value if $1 - F_k(z) < \pi_0$, which can happen if π_0 is close to 1, i.e. if the effect is zero for the majority of subsets. An estimator of the Fdr can be obtained as a by-product of the parameter estimation process, which is described in the next section.

5.3 PARAMETER ESTIMATION

5.3.1 Posterior Means and Variances

Let the prior distribution g depend on a parameter vector $\psi = (\psi_1, \ldots, \psi_M)$. For example for the single component normal prior, $\psi = (\eta, \tau)$. Let

$$f(z; \psi) = \frac{1}{\sigma} \int \phi\left(\frac{z-\theta}{\sigma}\right) g(\theta; \psi) d\theta \quad (5.13)$$

The maximum likelihood estimator $\hat{\psi}$ of ψ is then obtained from maximizing the log marginal likelihood

$$\ell(\psi; z) = \sum_{i=1}^{I} \log f_k(z; \psi)$$

where f_k denotes the marginal density of Z_k. In a second step one obtains estimators $\hat{\theta}_k(z)$ and $\hat{\sigma}_k^2(z)$ of $\theta_k(z)$ and $\sigma_k^2(z)$ from

$$\hat{\theta}_k(z) = z + \sigma_k^2 \frac{d \log f_k(z; \hat{\psi})}{dz},$$

$$\hat{\sigma}_k(z) = \sigma_k^2 \left[1 + \sigma_k^2 \frac{d^2 \log f_k(z; \hat{\psi})}{dz^2}\right].$$

This procedure ignores variability of $\hat{\psi}$ when it comes to variance estimation. A correction term can be obtained from the conditional mean squared error of prediction (CMSEP) for generalized linear mixed models (Booth and Hobert, 1998) that reads, in our situation,

$$\begin{aligned}\text{CMSEP}(\psi; z) &= E[\{\hat{\theta}_k(z) - \theta_k\}^2] \\ &= V[\theta_k | Z_k = z] + E[\{\hat{\theta}_k(z) - \theta_k(z)\}^2] \\ &= \sigma_k^2(z) + E[\{\hat{\theta}_k(z) - \theta_k(z)\}^2].\end{aligned}$$

Now

$$\hat{\theta}_k(z) - \theta_k(z)$$
$$= \sigma_k^2 \left[\frac{d \log f_k(z; \hat{\psi})}{dz} - \frac{d \log f_k(z; \psi)}{dz} \right] \quad (5.14)$$
$$\approx \sigma_k^2 \left[\sum_{m=1}^{K} \frac{\partial}{\partial \psi_m} \left(\frac{d \log f_k(z; \psi)}{dz} \right) (\hat{\psi}_m - \psi_m) \right]$$
$$(5.15)$$

and therefore

$$E[\{\hat{\theta}_k(z) - \theta_k(z)\}^2]$$
$$\approx \sigma_k^4 \left[\sum_{m=1}^{K} \sum_{l=1}^{K} \frac{\partial}{\partial \psi_m} \left(\frac{d \log f_k(z; \psi)}{dz} \right) \right.$$
$$\left. \times \frac{\partial}{\partial \psi_l} \left(\frac{d \log f_k(z; \psi)}{dz} \right) E[(\hat{\psi}_m - \psi_m)(\hat{\psi}_l - \psi_l)] \right].$$
$$(5.16)$$

The same approximation can be derived using the posterior distribution of ψ given Z (Kass and Steffey, 1989). To illustrate this equation we consider a one component normal prior for which $\psi = (\eta, \tau)$ and

$$\ell_k(\psi; z) = \frac{d \log f_k(z; \psi)}{dz} = -\frac{z - \eta}{\sigma_k^2 + \tau^2}$$

holds. In this case

$$\frac{\partial}{\partial \eta}\ell_k(\psi; z) = \frac{1}{\sigma_k^2 + \tau^2}, \quad \frac{\partial}{\partial \tau}\ell_k(\psi; z) = \frac{2\tau(z - \eta)}{(\sigma_k^2 + \tau^2)^2}.$$

Therefore

$$\hat{\theta}_k(z) - \theta_k(z) \approx \sigma_k^2 \left[\frac{\hat{\eta} - \eta}{\sigma_k^2 + \tau^2} + 2\tau \frac{z - \eta}{(\sigma_k^2 + \tau^2)^2}(\hat{\tau} - \tau) \right]$$

$$= (1 - \omega_k)[\hat{\eta} - \eta + 2\omega_k(z - \eta)(\hat{\tau} - \tau)/\tau]$$

and

$$E[\{\hat{\theta}_k(z) - \theta_k(z)\}^2]$$
$$\approx (1 - \omega_k)^2 V[\hat{\eta}] + 4[\omega_k(1 - \omega_k)(z - \eta)/\tau]^2 V[\hat{\tau}]$$
$$+ 4\omega_k(1 - \omega_k)((z - \eta)/\tau)\mathrm{Cov}[\hat{\eta}, \hat{\tau}]$$

and the left hand side can be estimated by plugging in parameter and variance/covariance estimates obtained from maximizing the marginal likelihood. Note that in the case $\hat{\tau}^2 \approx 0$ also $\hat{\omega} \approx 0$ and hence $\hat{\sigma}^2$ would be equal to $\hat{V}(\hat{\eta})$, the variance estimator of $\hat{\eta}$.

In the general case a maximum likelihood estimation requires the calculation of a complex integral. For the mixture prior the likelihood corresponding to the marginal distribution (5.7) simplifies to

$$\ell(\pi, \eta, \tau^2; z) = \sum_{k=1}^{K} \log \left\{ \sum_{j=0}^{J} \pi_j \phi_{kj}(z_k) \right\}. \quad (5.17)$$

Maximization of (5.17) can be achieved by using gradient methods. For many component priors one can start off with an expectation maximization algorithm (Dempster et al., 1977) to improve the likelihood to a certain extent and take the final estimates as starting values for a gradient based optimizer to finish off. Matters simplify for the standard hierarchical model

$$\ell(\eta_0, \tau_0^2; z) = \sum_{k=1}^{K} \log\{\phi_{k0}(z_k)\} \quad (5.18)$$

which can be fitted in a straightforward manner without causing major convergence problems.

5.3.2 Estimation Bias

It was shown that under the conditions of Corollary 5.1 the posterior variance of the effects in a subgroup is smaller under a hierarchical model as compared to a per group analysis. The question arises: what happens to the bias of $\hat{\theta}_k(z)$ as an estimator of θ_k? Since the latter is considered random, an extended definition of bias is required. As often done in selection problems, we define the bias of $\hat{\theta}$ as an estimator of θ as in Rosenkranz (2014)

$$B(\hat{\theta}, \theta) = E[\hat{\theta} - \theta]. \quad (5.19)$$

Note that with this definition, $B(Z_k, \theta_k) = 0$.

Corollary 5.3: *The EB estimator is consistent and asymptotically unbiased in the sense of (5.19).*

Proof: For the EB estimator it follows that

$$B(\hat{\theta}_k(Z_k), \theta_k) = E[\hat{\theta}_k(Z_k) - \theta_k(Z_k)] + E[\theta_k(Z_k) - \theta_k].$$

The second term is zero because of

$$E[\theta_k(Z_k) - \theta_k]$$

$$= E[Z_k - \theta_k] + E\left[\sigma_k^2 \frac{d \log f_k(z)}{dz}\bigg|_{z=Z_k}\right]$$

$$= \sigma_k^2 \int f'_k(z) dz$$

$$= \int \left[\int \frac{z-\theta}{\sigma_k} \phi\left(\frac{z-\theta}{\sigma_k}\right) dz\right] g(\theta) d\theta = 0.$$

Since the maximum likelihood estimator $\hat{\psi}$ is consistent, it follows from (5.15) that $\hat{\theta}_k(z) \to \theta_k(z)$ almost surely for $K \to \infty$.

5.3.3 Selection Bias

The Fdr allows selecting only those units for which the risk of false discovery is low. The question then arises how to estimate the parameters for the selected units. It is fairly obvious that the per group estimator is biased after selection.

Corollary 5.4: *Assume that a subgroup is selected if the respective $Z_k > z$. Then*

$$E[Z_k - \theta_k | Z_k > z] = \sigma_k^2 f_k(z) / \Pr[Z_k > z]$$

while

$$E[\hat{\theta}_k(Z_k) - \theta_k | Z_k > z] \to 0 \quad \text{for } K \to \infty.$$

Proof: Observe that

$$E[\theta_k | Z_k > z] = E[E[\theta_k | Z_k] | Z_k > z]$$
$$= E[\theta_k(Z_k) | Z_k > z]$$

and

$$E\left[\frac{d \log f(Z_k)}{dz} | Z_k > z\right] = \frac{1}{\Pr[Z_k > z]} \int_z^\infty f'(t) dt$$
$$= -\frac{f(z)}{\Pr[Z_k > z]}.$$

Then

$$E[Z_k - \theta_k | Z_k > z] = E[Z_k - \theta(Z_k) | Z_k > z]$$
$$= \sigma^2 f(z) / \Pr[Z_k > z]$$

and

$$E[\hat{\theta}_k(Z_k) - \theta_k | Z_k > z]$$
$$= E[\hat{\theta}_k(Z_k) - \theta_i(Z_k) | Z_k > z] \to 0$$

since $\hat{\theta}_k(Z_k) \to \theta_k(Z_k)$ almost surely from the previous corollary. The following simulation gives an idea of the extent selection bias in the original estimator can be reduced. We consider a situation with 20 subsets and a two component prior with an atom at 0 and a normal component with a mixture probability of 0.5. More precisely, for each of 10 000 simulations we generated $K = 20$ indicators with $X_k \sim \text{Bern}(1 - \pi_0)$ for $\pi_0 = 0.5$. For $X_k = 0$ we set $\theta_k = 0$, otherwise we randomly drew θ_k from a $N(1, \tau^2)$ distribution with $\tau = 0.25, 0.5, 1$. Eventually we generated Z_k with distribution $N(\theta_k, 0.5^2)$. Next we maximized the marginal likelihood of Z to obtain estimates $\hat{\pi}_0$, $\hat{\eta}_1$ and $\hat{\tau}_1^2$ and calculated the EB estimates $\hat{\theta}_{2k}(z)$. To see what happens if the analysis model is mis-specified we fitted a hierarchical model with a single component prior to obtain $\hat{\eta}$, $\hat{\tau}^2$ and $\hat{\theta}_{1k}$. Finally we selected from each simulation the units with values $Z_k > 2$. The boxplots for the means of $Z_k - \theta_k$, $\hat{\theta}_{1k}(Z_k) - \theta_k$ and $\hat{\theta}_{2k}(Z_k) - \theta_k$ from the selected and unselected data are shown in Figure 5.1.

On the full data, the estimator Z is unbiased, while there is some tiny bias in the EB estimates. Clearly the estimator from the correct model

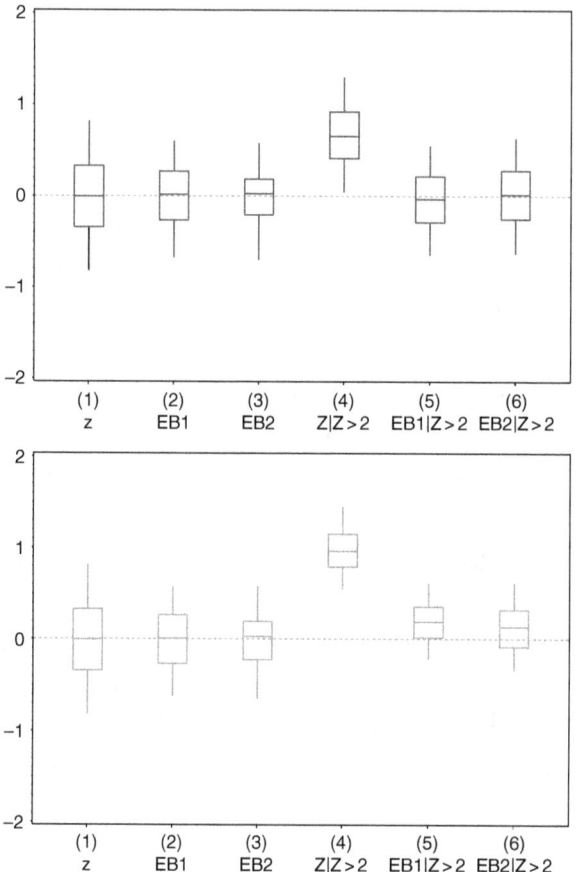

Figure 5.1 Box plots of the means of the bias estimates from all 10 000 simulated datasets (1–3) and from the data with Z > 2 (4–6). Data were simulated from a two component prior with $\pi_0 = 0.5$, $\eta_1 = 1$, $\sigma = 0.5$, $\tau_1 = 0.25, 0.5, 1$ (upper left to lower panel) and $K = 20$. Biases of the original estimates (Z), empirical Bayes estimates from an analysis with single component prior (EB1) and the true model (EB2) are shown. (For details see text.)

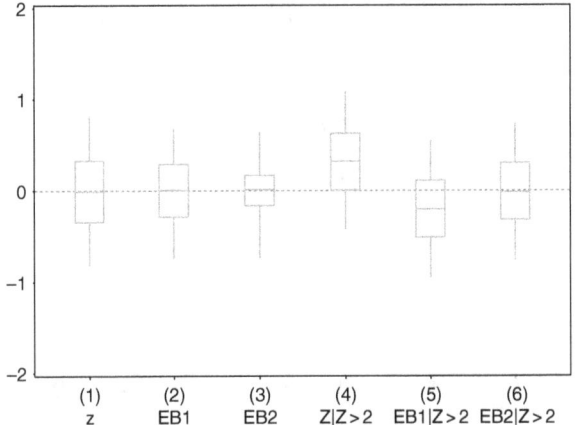

Figure 5.1 (*Continued*)

has the smallest variability, however, also the one based on the single component prior is less variable then the group wise estimator which is in agreement with Stein's result (Stein, 1956). The EB estimators assuming a one or two mixture prior are doing a good job in terms of selection bias reduction as compared to the raw estimates if $\tau = \sigma = 0.5$. For $\tau = 0.25 < \sigma = 0.5$, they correct quite well. For $\tau = 1 > \sigma = 0.5$, the analysis using a two component prior corrects remarkably well while the model using the single component prior starts over-correcting for selection bias.

A rationale for this behavior of the analysis relying on the wrong model is as follows. Let $\theta_1(z)$ and $\theta_2(z)$ be the expectation of the posterior distribution of θ under the single and two component model, respectively, then using notation from Section 5.2.2,

$$\Delta(z) = \theta_1(z) - \theta_2(z) = \omega_J z + (1 - \omega_J)\eta_J \\ - Q_1[\omega_1 z + (1 - \omega_1)\eta_1] \quad (5.20)$$

with

$$\eta_J = (1 - \pi_0)\eta_1,$$
$$\tau_J^2 = \pi_0 \eta_J^2 + (1 - \pi_0)[\tau_1^2 + (\eta_1 - \eta_J)^2]$$

and

$$\omega_1 = \frac{\tau_1^2}{\tau_1^2 + \sigma^2}, \quad \omega_J = \frac{\tau_J^2}{\tau_J^2 + \sigma^2}.$$

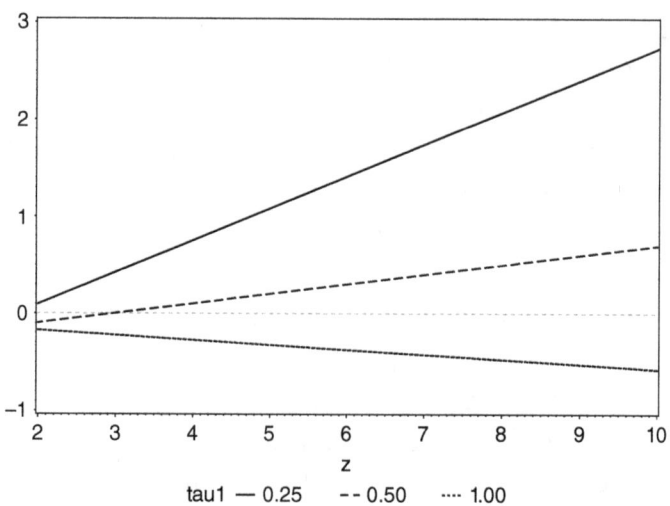

Figure 5.2 Differences between the posterior means of a model with a single prior and with the true two component prior (5.20) as a function of z. (For details see text.)

A plot of $\Delta(z)$ for different values of τ_1 is shown in the bottom right panel of Figure 5.2. For $\tau_1 = 1$, $\Delta(z) < 0$ for $z > 2$, implying a negative bias of $\hat{\theta}_1$ as an estimator of θ.

5.4 CASE STUDIES

This section illustrates the applicability of the modeling and estimation procedures described earlier to some well known datasets from the literature. Note that all examples are analyzed using the naive variance estimator not correcting for variability of the parameter estimates for the prior. While simplifying calculations it still preserves relevant aspects when comparing models based on single component and mixture priors. In particular the goodness-of-fit measures are not affected. In the first example the analysis suggest that a simple hierarchical model may suffice while in the other two the mixture prior provides a better fit than the simple model. Interestingly, the first dataset includes almost three times as many groups than the second one.

5.4.1 The Toxoplasmosis Dataset

This data stems from a study of toxoplasmosis in El Salvador where sera was obtained from 5171 individuals of varying ages from 36 cities (Remington et al., 1970). From the data provided in that paper toxoplasmosis prevalence rates Z_k for each city were calculated. The prevalence rates have the form (observed−expected)/expected, with observed being the number of positives for a city and expected the number of positives for the same city based on an indirect standardization of prevalence due to age distribution in a city. The variances σ_k were derived from binomial considerations and differ because of unequal sample sizes.

The dataset was re-analyzed in Efron and Morris (1975) to illustrate data analysis using empirical Bayes methodology. They fitted the model

$$Z_k|\theta_k \sim N(\theta_k, \sigma_k^2), \quad \theta_k|\tau \sim N(0, \tau^2)$$

thereby fixing the prior mean at zero. In the following we fit a hierarchical model with a more general single component prior $N(\eta, \tau^2)$, and a mixture prior with three components including a null component. The marginal likelihood was maximized with a Newton–Raphson optimizer with a grid search for starting values for the more complex model. The results are shown in Table 5.1.

The likelihood increases with model complexity as expected. When the likelihood is penalized for complexity, the model with the one component prior provides the best fit while the BIC for the three component model is substantially higher. Likewise the standard errors of the parameter estimates for the most complex model are rather

Table 5.1 Estimates of the model parameters for the toxoplasmosis data

Prior	One component	Three components including a null
Parameter estimates (standard errors)	$\hat{\eta}_0 = -0.018(0.023)$ $\hat{\tau}_0 = 0.111(0.021)$	$\hat{\eta}_1 = -0.118(0.231)$ $\hat{\eta}_2 = 0.070(0.182)$ $\hat{\tau}_1 = 0.108(0.128)$ $\hat{\tau}_2 = 0.072(0.072)$ $\hat{\pi}_1 = 0.420(0.713)$ $\hat{\pi}_2 = 0.377(0.957)$
$-2 \log ll$	-32.0	-33.0
AIC	-28.0	-21.0
BIC	-24.8	-11.5

large. Furthermore introducing more components in the model does not result in substantially different empirical Bayes estimates in cities with a lower or higher than expected prevalence, as illustrated in Figure 5.3. Hence, as suggested by the data, the one component prior seems to be adequate.

5.4.2 The BCG Dataset

Next we consider a meta analysis to quantify the efficacy of the Bacillus Calmette–Guérin (BCG) vaccination in the prevention of tuberculosis (TB) (Colditz et al., 1994). Studies were selected from the literature. Eventually 70 articles were reviewed for method of vaccine allocation, equivalent surveillance and follow-up for recipient and

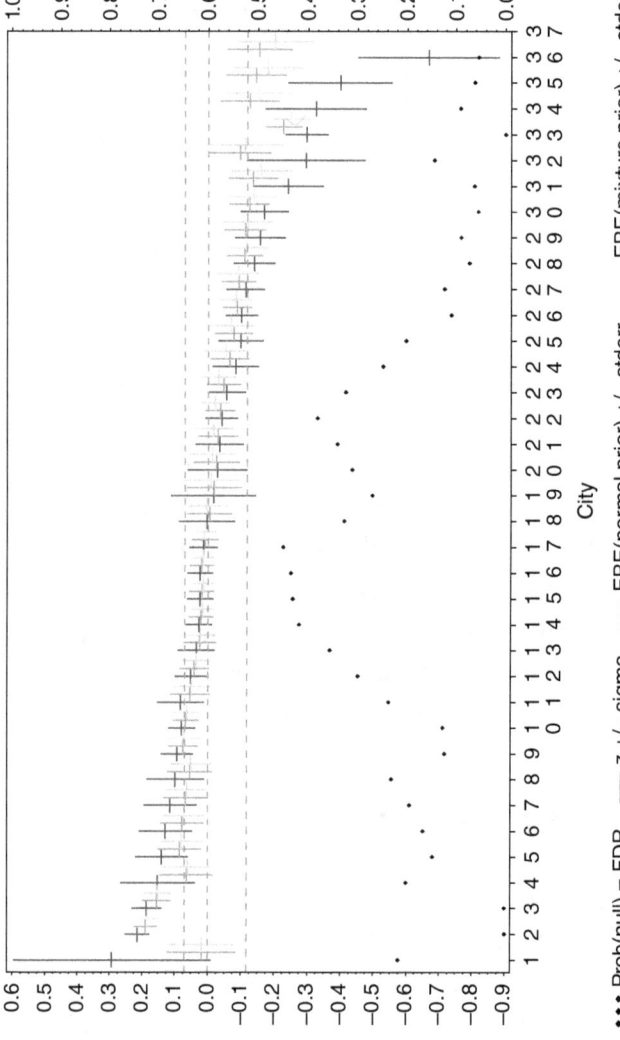

Figure 5.3 Original estimates (blue) and empirical Bayes estimates for the single prior (red) and the mixture prior (green) for the toxoplasmosis data.

concurrent control groups, and outcome measures of TB cases. These criteria were summarized in a validity score. Thirteen prospective studies with a control group were selected, some of which were randomized trials while in others vaccination was assigned alternately or systematically to individuals. This data was analyzed using the DerSimomian and Laird random effects model (DerSimonian and Laird, 1986). The data was re-analyzed in the literature to illustrate EB estimation (van Houwelingen, 2014) or meta regression (Simmonds and Higgins, 2016), among others.

The summary data sorted by increasing log-odds ratios or decreasing vaccine efficacy is presented in Table 5.2. The majority of 10 studies demonstrate an effect in favor of BCG, in one smaller study (number 13) the effect was reversed; however, more importantly, two very large studies (numbers 11 and 12) show virtually no protecting effect. This indicates that a one-component hierarchical model may not adequately describe the data. From a medical standpoint an explanation is requested for the reason behind this dichotomy of effects.

We fitted hierarchical models with a one- and a two-component prior with an atom at zero since there is little indication for a negative impact of vaccination. Parameter estimates and fit statistics are provided in Table 5.3. The results from the one component prior model are very close to those obtained earlier in Colditz et al. (1994), Simmonds and Higgins (2016), van Houwelingen (2014).

Table 5.2 BCG data

Trial	Vaccinated		Not vaccinated		ln(OR)	Latitude	Allocation
	Disease	No disease	Disease	No disease			
1	6	300	29	274	−1.67	55	R
2	8	2537	10	619	−1.63	19	R
3	62	13536	248	12619	−1.46	52	R
4	17	1699	65	1600	−1.40	42	S
5	3	228	11	209	−1.39	42	R
6	180	1361	372	1079	−0.96	44	A
7	4	119	11	128	−0.94	44	R
8	29	7470	45	7232	−0.47	27	R
9	186	50448	141	27197	−0.34	18	S
10	33	5036	47	5761	−0.22	13	A
11	27	16886	29	17825	−0.02	33	S
12	505	87886	499	87892	**0.01**	13	R
13	5	2493	3	2338	0.45	33	S

Table 5.3 Estimates of the model parameters for the BCG data

Prior	One component	Two components including a null
Parameter estimates (stderr)	$\hat{\eta}_1 = -0.742(0.179)$ $\hat{\tau}_1 = 0.550(0.142)$	$\hat{\eta}_2 = -0.962(0.223)$ $\hat{\tau}_2 = 0.468(0.160)$ $\hat{\pi}_0 = 0.238(0.175)$
$-2 \log ll$	26.1	23.2
AIC	30.1	29.2
BIC	31.3	30.9

The model based on the mixture prior enables a better fit, both in terms of a higher likelihood and in regard to the penalized goodness-of-fit measures. The effect estimates per study are shown in Figure 5.4. Studies 11 and 12 belong to the null set with high posterior probability (Fdr > 0.7 or > 0.9) with an almost vanishing standard error for the effect in study 12.

An explanation for the absence of efficacy in some of the biggest studies provided in the original paper refers to the geographic latitude of the study centers (see Table 5.2) and a validity score mentioned earlier. Jointly they explain 66% of the between trial variation. Individually, latitude explains 41%, validity 30%. In a meta analysis of case control studies, which is not shown here, the only covariate explaining a big part of the between trial variability (36%) is data validity (Colditz et al., 1994). Latitude was also considered

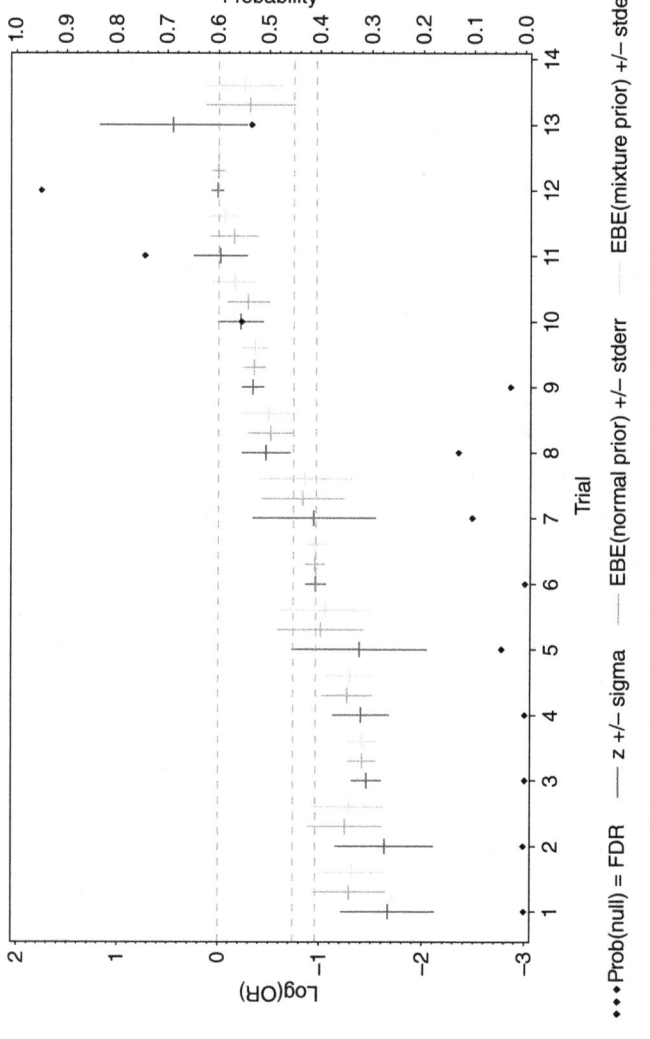

Figure 5.4 Original estimates (blue) and empirical Bayes estimates for the single prior (red) and the mixture prior (green) for the BCG data.

as a covariate in a meta regression of the BCG data resulting in an estimated 0.97 change of effect per degree latitude with a 95% confidence interval of (0.96 − 0.98) (Simmonds and Higgins, 2016) indicating that a one-component prior may not appropriately describe the data. Whether latitude is really the root cause of between trial variability or at best a proxy for another unknown factor cannot be decided from the data. Another explanation could be the decreasing prevalence of the disease over the years or in some regions.

5.4.3 The Prostate Cancer Dataset

In this investigation, 6033 genes were studied in each of 102 men, 50 healthy controls and 52 prostate cancer patients (Singh et al., 2002). For the following calculations independence of the gene expression levels was assumed, which may not be the case for micro-array data in general.

Let T_k be the two sample t-statistic comparing the averages of the gene expression levels of healthy subjects versus cancer subjects for gene k. T_k is transformed to a normal scale such that

$$Z_k = \Phi^{-1}(F_{100}(T_k)),$$

where F_n denotes the cdf of a t-distribution with n degrees of freedom. Most of the genes are presumably neutral in regard to prostate cancer while some may be prognostic. To figure this out we assume a single component prior to start with,

Table 5.4 Estimates of the model parameters for the prostate cancer data

Prior	One component	Three components including a null
Parameter estimates (standard errors)	$\hat{\eta} = 0.003(0.015)$ $\hat{\tau} = 0.537(0.022)$	$\hat{\eta}_1 = 1.832(0.751)$ $\hat{\eta}_2 = -2.040(0.545)$ $\hat{\tau}_1 = 0.695(0.473)$ $\hat{\tau}_2 = 0.203(1.061)$ $\hat{\pi}_1 = 0.038(0.023)$ $\hat{\pi}_2 = 0.032(0.016)$
$-2 \log ll$	18649	18574
AIC	18653	18586
BIC	18667	18626

and a three component prior with a null case component.

The results of the analysis are shown in Table 5.4. Clearly the one component prior is inferior in terms of likelihood and model fit as measured by AIC or BIC. For the three component prior, the proportion of unrelated genes is estimated to be 93%, which leaves us with about 422 interesting ones.

The upper part of Figure 5.5 shows the estimators Z_k and $\theta_k(z)$ and their standard errors for each gene and the single component prior. For better visibility we have ordered Z_k from smallest to largest and re-numbered the genes accordingly. As expected there is a substantial shrinkage for the extreme Z_k. Furthermore, since $\sigma_k = 1$ for all genes, the standard errors of the EB estimates

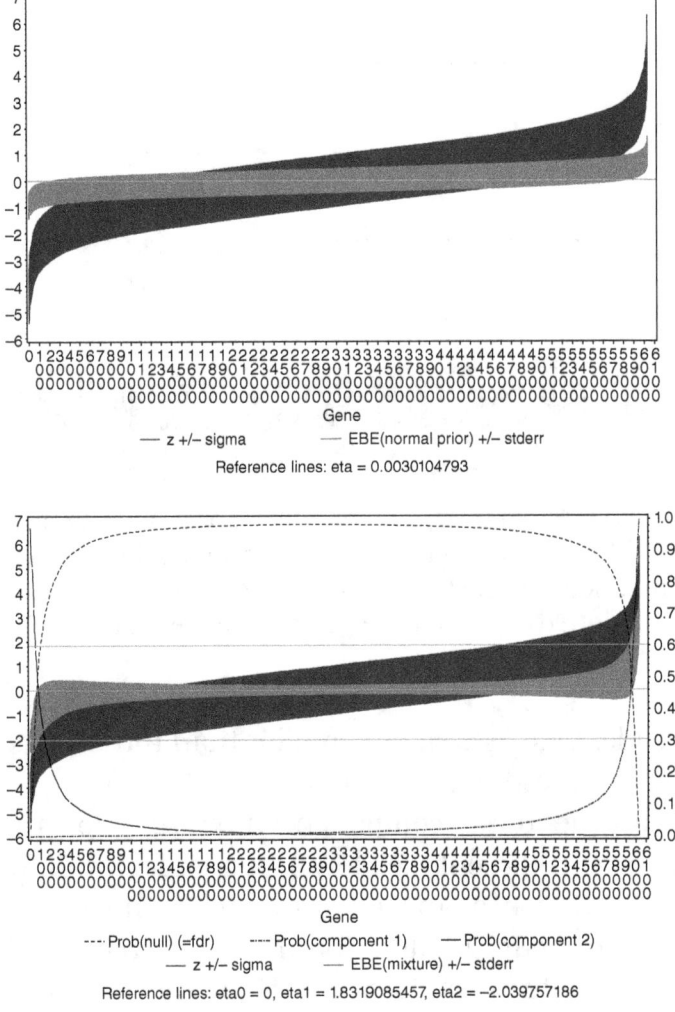

Figure 5.5 Original estimates (dark gray) and empirical Bayes estimates for a single component prior (light gray, upper graph) and a mixture prior (light gray, lower graph).

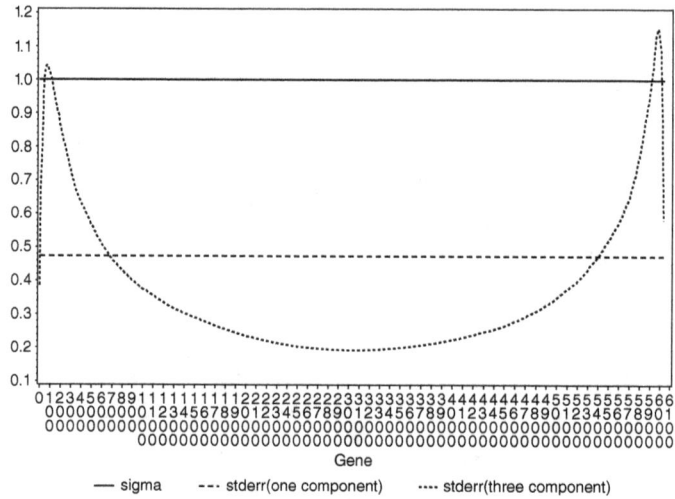

Figure 5.6 Standard errors of the original estimates (solid line) and empirical Bayes estimates for the one component (dashed line) and three component mixture prior (dotted curve) for the prostate cancer data.

are identical as well but smaller than those of the gene-wise estimates.

For the three component mixture prior the picture is different (see lower part of Figure 5.5). The variance of the EB estimator is no longer constant, but smallest for medium sized Z_k. A graph of the standard errors of the estimates is drawn in Figure 5.6 showing that the one component empirical Bayes estimator is uniformly less variable than the gene-wise estimator while the three component prior leads to an estimator with lowest standard error for a range of Z_k but also highest standard errors accounting for the uncertainty to which component Z_k belongs.

Table 5.5 Estimates and standard error of the gene expression difference by the original z-values and the EB estimators with a one and three component prior for genes with fdr ≤ 0.1

Gene	Z	EB1(SE)	EB3(SE)
1	−4.42	−0.99(0.47)	−2.08(0.39)
2	−4.33	−0.97(0.47)	−2.07(0.41)
3	−4.29	−0.96(0.47)	−2.06(0.43)
4	−4.14	−0.93(0.47)	−2.03(0.48)
5	−3.88	−0.87(0.47)	−1.96(0.59)
6	−3.88	−0.87(0.47)	−1.95(0.59)
7	−3.84	−0.86(0.47)	−1.94(0.61)
8	−3.82	−0.85(0.47)	−1.93(0.62)
6019	3.69	0.83(0.47)	2.20(0.90)
6020	3.72	0.84(0.47)	2.23(0.88)
6021	3.88	0.87(0.47)	2.34(0.82)
6022	3.97	0.89(0.47)	2.40(0.78)
6023	3.98	0.89(0.47)	2.41(0.78)
6024	3.98	0.89(0.47)	2.41(0.78)
6025	4.10	0.92(0.47)	2.48(0.74)
6026	4.12	0.93(0.47)	2.49(0.73)
6027	4.14	0.93(0.47)	2.50(0.73)
6028	4.19	0.94(0.47)	2.52(0.71)
6029	4.25	0.95(0.47)	2.55(0.70)
6030	4.40	0.99(0.47)	2.62(0.66)
6031	4.47	1.00(0.47)	2.66(0.65)
6032	4.83	1.08(0.47)	2.80(0.60)
6033	5.29	1.19(0.47)	2.96(0.58)

Table 5.5 shows the z-values and the EB estimates for the gene expression difference between sick and healthy subjects. Those genes with an fdr less than 10% as determined from the three component mixture model are adding up to 23

of 6033. As expected, the z-values have to be way above the common critical level of 1.96 to be selected. The feedback to a scientist having conducted this study is that about 21 of these 23 genes are potentially promising candidates for identifying subjects with prostate cancer and that confirming investigations can focus on this subset. The table shows also the estimates obtained from the inadequate one component model with its rather drastic extent of shrinkage.

5.5 CONCLUDING REMARKS

We have investigated generalizations of the often applied normal–normal hierarchical model to account for situations where the distribution of the group parameters is non-unique or in other words where the group parameters are not completely exchangeable. Empirical Bayes methodology has been used to obtain parameter estimates and standard errors. While presenting the methodology, some theoretical results regarding estimation and selection bias have been established. These results have been complimented with simulations illustrating the impact of choosing the wrong model.

Generalizing the prior in a hierarchical model by introducing mixtures of normal distributions and atoms may not uniformly increase both precision and accuracy over the normal–normal model. The

Concluding Remarks 125

reason is the additional uncertainty as to which mixture component a group belongs. In case this uncertainty is small, i.e. the posterior probability for a group to belong to a component is either close to 0 or 1, the variance of the EB estimators can be much smaller than for the one component prior. For groups where this probability is close to one half, it can exceed the variability of the group-wise estimator. For a one component prior, there is no such uncertainty and the EB estimate is less variable than the within group estimator for each group.

Fitting a multi-component prior requires more information on the data side, otherwise the parameter estimates for different components of the marginal distribution may become non-identifiable. This manifests numerically by obtaining identical parameter estimates for different components or zero posterior probabilities for all but one component, resulting in singular covariance matrix estimates. More general models produce a larger likelihood, but the goodness-of-fit measures accounting for model complexity may deteriorate, as illustrated in one of the examples.

The question of how many components are actually required remains an issue. In many cases plausible reasoning will provide a good starting point. This can include statistical as well as scientific considerations. In the prostate cancer example it was obvious that only a fraction of the investigated genes has an impact. Goodness-of-fit measures like those used in the examples provide some guidance. Simulations presented showed that depending on the circumstances EB methods can be advantageous for analyses concerning about 20 groups, but it would be difficult to come up with precise criteria since this depends on the (unknown) effects and the within and between group variability. Covariates, where available, can be helpful in assessing the plausibility of certain model assumptions. The Fdr can support identification of relevant subsets, the corresponding estimates will be less biased than standard estimates.

However, we would generally refrain from using any results from exploratory analyses at face value without a challenge for scientific plausibility or confirmation in follow-up investigations. Many results from subgroup analyses in clinical studies have never been corroborated by additional evidence and the majority of those that have, could not be confirmed (Wallach et al., 2017). Using subgroup analyses in a drug development and regulatory context requires specific considerations (Grouin et al., 2005).

The EB approach has the advantage that the priors do not have to be specified, but that the prior parameters are estimated from the marginal likelihood of the data. The latter can be maximized by standard optimization procedures. On the other hand, one has to take care not to underestimate variances of the EB estimators. A Bayesian framework would avoid the latter, since the variability information is reflected in the posterior distribution. The assumptions on the prior influences the analysis results as well, in particular for small number of groups, which in turn could be used to determine the dependence of the results on the assumptions on the prior. For more discussions on the future of Bayesian and/or empirical Bayesian methodology (see Carlin and Louis, 2000, 2009).

In theory, Robbins' theorem (Robbins, 1956) enables one to perform an empirical Bayes estimation without knowing the prior or the distributional class it belongs to in the case where the group estimators are independently identically distributed, as in the prostate cancer example. This can be more generally achieved for Wald statistics (Efron, 2011). Precision and accuracy of this so-called non-parametric EB approach would need to be investigated further.

6

Selection Bias in Regression

No history can be a faithful mirror. If it were, it would be as long and as dull as life itself. It must be a selection, and, being a selection, must inevitably be biased.

Thomas Ernest Hulme (1883-1917)

6.1 INTRODUCTION

For quite some time parameter estimation after variable or model selection was performed as if the final model was selected without reference to the data. However, using the same data for choosing a model and estimating parameters may induce selection bias, i.e. an overoptimism in the estimates. In this section we discuss a proposal for estimation after selection based on re-sampling.

Re-sampling methods have proven to constitute valuable statistical methods to estimate the variance or the bias of a parameter estimator in cases where these estimates cannot be obtained in closed form. The bootstrap developed in Efron (1979) has become most popular in this context. An introduction to the latter can be found in Efron and Tibshirani (1986, 1993).

Application of the bootstrap has been extended to tackle issues of model selection. When the same selection procedure as for the original study is used in an ideal validation trial, e.g., on a population defined by the same eligibility criteria, then ideally (nearly) the same variables should be selected, resulting in a (nearly) identical model. Analyzing survival data, Chen and George (1985) applied the same selection procedure to 100 bootstrap samples of the original data. They could reproduce the original model only in 2% of replications, providing some indication of the instability of the final model. However, the inclusion frequencies of five of the variables from the original model ranged between 64% and 82%, whereas the frequencies were much smaller for variables not included in the original model, suggesting that the most relevant variables had been selected. Consequently the inclusion frequencies may be used as an indicator for the importance of a variable or even in a variable selection strategy (Sauerbrei and Schumacher, 1992; Sauerbrei, 1999).

The idea of applying the same selection criteria to bootstrap samples of the original data was pursued further by Breiman (1996) who realized that averaging or aggregating predictors across bootstrap samples (so-called bootstrap aggregating or bagging for short) can reduce the variability of predictors. This is particularly true for neural nets, classification and regression trees, and subset selection in linear regression. Bagging was further investigated from a theoretical point of view in Bühlmann and Yu (2002).

Efron (2014) provided a variance estimator of bagged predictors that can be used to obtain confidence intervals after selection. If the model selection process is unknown the best possible approach is to consider all possible selections (Berk et al., 2013), resulting in very conservative confidence intervals. A bias correction of an effect estimator after selection based on re-sampling is described in Rosenkranz (2014, 2016).

6.2 CORRECTION FOR SELECTION BIAS

Let $\mathcal{L} = \{L_1, \ldots, L_N\}$ be independently identically distributed random variables (the learning dataset) and θ a parameter of interest with estimator $\hat{\theta} = t(\mathcal{L})$. For example if $L_n = Y_n$ (a scalar) and $\theta = E[Y_n]$, then $\hat{\theta} = t(\mathbf{Y}) = \frac{1}{N}\sum_{n=1}^{N} Y_n$. In a regression context, let $L_n = (Y_n, \mathbf{X}_n)$ with

$Y_n \sim N(\mathbf{X}_n \theta, \sigma^2)$. Then with $\mathbf{X} = (\mathbf{X}_1, \ldots, \mathbf{X}_N)$, $\hat{\theta} = t(\mathbf{Y}, \mathbf{X}) = (\mathbf{X}'\mathbf{X})^{-1}\mathbf{X}'\mathbf{Y}$. In either situation, the estimators are unbiased and their standard error can be obtained in a straightforward manner.

A generic estimator of the standard error of an estimate can be obtained as follows: draw a series of $b = 1, \ldots, B$ bootstrap samples $\mathcal{L}_b^* = \{L_{b1}^*, \ldots, L_{bN}^*\}$, each consisting of N draws with replacement from the learning set $\mathcal{L}$, yielding bootstrap estimates $\hat{\theta}_b^* = t(\mathcal{L}_b^*)$. The bootstrap estimate of standard error is the standard deviation of the bootstrap replications

$$\hat{\sigma}_B^* = \sqrt{\sum_{b=1}^{B} (\hat{\theta}_b^* - \hat{\theta}_B^*)^2 / (B-1)} \qquad (6.1)$$

where $\hat{\theta}_B^* = \sum_{b=1}^{B} \hat{\theta}_b^* / B$ (Efron and Tibshirani, 1993). $\hat{\theta}_B^*$ is called the *aggregated* or *bagged* (bootstrap aggregated) estimator. Its importance will become clear later.

The bias of an estimator $\hat{\theta}$ of a parameter θ is defined as

$$B(\hat{\theta}, \theta) = E[\hat{\theta}] - \theta.$$

The bootstrap can also deliver a generic estimate for the bias of an estimator, namely (Efron and Tibshirani, 1993)

$$\hat{B}_B^*(\hat{\theta}, \theta) = \hat{\theta}_B^* - \hat{\theta}. \qquad (6.2)$$

Can the bootstrap also help in providing an estimator of selection bias?

Assume that the data $\mathcal{L}$ are divided into K groups $\mathcal{L}_k$, $k = 1, \ldots, K$. For each group a parameter θ_k is to be estimated by an estimator $\hat{\theta}_k$. Define selection functions $u_k : \mathcal{L} \to \{0, 1\}$ such that $\mathcal{L}_k$ is selected if $u_k = 1$. As an example consider $u_k = 1$ if $\hat{\theta}_k = \max(\hat{\theta}_1, \ldots \hat{\theta}_K)$. The bias of $\hat{\theta}_k$ conditional on $u_k = 1$, the *selection bias*, is then given by

$$B(\hat{\theta}_k, \theta_k | u_k = 1) = E[\hat{\theta}_k | u_k = 1] - \theta_k$$
$$= \frac{E[u_k \hat{\theta}_k]}{E[u_k]} - \theta_k.$$

For a bootstrap sample $\mathcal{L}_b^*$ of $\mathcal{L}$ let $u_{bk}^* = u_k(\mathcal{L}_b^*)$ and $\hat{\theta}_{bk}^* = \hat{\theta}_k(\mathcal{L}_b^*)$. Then the bootstrap bias estimator after selection is given by (Rosenkranz, 2014)

$$\hat{B}^*(\hat{\theta}_k, \theta_k | u_k = 1) = \frac{\sum_{b=1}^{B} u_{bk}^* \hat{\theta}_{bk}^*}{\sum_{b=1}^{B} u_{bk}^*} - \hat{\theta}_k$$

and the bias corrected estimator by

$$\check{\theta}_k^* = 2\hat{\theta}_k - \frac{\sum_{b=1}^{B} u_{bk}^* \hat{\theta}_{bk}^*}{\sum_{b=1}^{B} u_{bk}^*}. \quad (6.3)$$

In other words, the bias correction is the mean of the parameter estimates from bootstrap samples where subgroup k has been selected.

The selection functions u_k depend on the *entire* dataset, not just on data from subgroup k. The proportion of bootstrap samples where $\mathcal{L}_k$ is selected,

$$\hat{p}_k^* = \frac{1}{B} \sum_{k=1}^{K} u_{bk}^*$$

provides an estimate of the (un)certainty that subgroup $\mathcal{L}_k$ has been correctly selected given the data $\mathcal{L}$. One can replace $\hat{\theta}_k$ in (6.3) by the aggregated estimator

$$\hat{\theta}_k^* = \sum_{b=1}^{B} \hat{\theta}_{bk}^*/B \qquad (6.4)$$

to obtain

$$\tilde{\theta}_k^* = \frac{1}{B} \sum_{b=1}^{B} \hat{\theta}_{bk}^* \left(2 - \frac{u_{bk}^*}{\hat{p}_k^*}\right). \qquad (6.5)$$

$\tilde{\theta}_k^*$ is a weighted mean of $\hat{\theta}_{bk}^*$ with weights $2 - u_{bk}^*/\hat{p}_k^*$ such that

$$2(1 - \hat{p}_k^*) + \hat{p}_k^*(2 - 1/\hat{p}_k^*) = 1$$

i.e. the estimates from each subgroup get an average weight of 1, but those from non-selected subgroups are up-weighted by a factor of 2 while estimates from selected subgroups are down-weighted by a factor of $2 - 1/\hat{p}_k^*$. If subgroup k is selected for all bootstrap samples, all weights equal 1 and (6.5) is identical to (6.4) and no correction for selection bias occurs. If subgroup k is selected for half of the bootstrap samples, the estimate for that group is the mean of the estimates of the samples where k was not selected.

Correction for Selection Bias

Which of the estimators (6.3) or (6.5) should one prefer? Using an argument similar to that in Breiman (1996) one can show that the mean squared error (MSE) of the latter is smaller for a sufficiently large number of bootstrap samples (Rosenkranz, 2016).

Theorem 6.1: $MSE[\tilde{\theta}_k^*] \leq MSE[\check{\theta}_k^*]$.

Proof: Let E^* denote the expectation under the "ideal bootstrap" where $B = N^N$ equals the number of all possible choices of bootstrap samples each having probability $1/B$. Define

$$\overline{\theta}_k^* = \frac{\sum_{b=1}^{B} u_{bk}^* \hat{\theta}_{bk}^*}{\sum_{b=1}^{B} u_{bk}^*}.$$

Applying Jensen's inequality it follows that

$$E^*[(\theta_k - (2\hat{\theta}_k - \overline{\theta}_k^*))^2] = \theta_k^2 - 2\theta_k E^*[2\hat{\theta}_k - \overline{\theta}_k^*] + E^*[(2\hat{\theta}_k - \overline{\theta}_k^*)^2]$$
$$\geq \theta_k^2 - 2\theta_k E^*[2\hat{\theta}_k - \overline{\theta}_k^*] + E^*[2\hat{\theta}_k - \overline{\theta}_k^*]^2$$
$$= (\theta_k - E^*[2\hat{\theta}_k - \overline{\theta}_k^*])^2$$
$$= (\theta_k - (2\hat{\theta}_k^* - \overline{\theta}_k^*))^2.$$

Taking the expectation over the distribution of the data on each side completes the proof.

The (theoretical) gain in precision depends on the difference

$$E^*[(2\hat{\theta}_k - \overline{\theta}_k^*)^2] - E^*[2\hat{\theta}_k - \overline{\theta}_k^*]^2.$$

For the inequality above to hold in practice, B has to be sufficiently large. The re-sampling method described can be used to correct for selection bias regardless of the selection procedure.

6.3 VARIANCE ESTIMATION

Eventually, to assess the variability of the bias reduced estimator of the selected subgroup, we need to know its variance and an estimator thereof. A simple approach would be to estimate the variance from the data of the selected subgroup as if no selection had taken place. Such an approach would ignore the additional uncertainty introduced by selection and would therefore potentially underestimate variability.

Another approach could be a second level of bootstrapping. Re-sampling from $\mathcal{L}_b^*$ would yield a collection of replications $\mathcal{L}_{bc}^*$ from which one could calculate $\hat{\theta}_b^* = \sum_{c=1}^B \hat{\theta}_{bc}^*/B$ for $b = 1, \ldots, B$ to obtain the bootstrap standard deviation from (6.1). However, this brute force approach would require an enormous number of recalculations. Efron (2014) proposed the *infinitesimal jackknife estimator* that uses only the original B bootstrap replications.

Theorem 6.2: Let $N_{bn}^* = \#\{j; L_{bj}^* = L_n\}$ be the number of elements of $\mathcal{L}_b^*$ equaling the original data point

L_n. Then for the ideal bootstrap with $B = N^N$

$$\tilde{V}^* = \sum_{n=1}^{N} C^*(N^*_{bn}, \theta^*_b))^2 \qquad (6.6)$$

i.e. the sum of the squared bootstrap covariances between N^*_{bn} and θ^*_b. The ideal estimate (6.6) can be approximated with

$$\tilde{V}^*_B = \frac{1}{B^2} \sum_{n=1}^{N} \left[\sum_{b=1}^{B} (N^*_{bn} - 1)(\hat{\theta}^*_b - \hat{\theta}^*_B) \right]^2. \qquad (6.7)$$

Let

$$\hat{V}^*_B = \frac{1}{B} \sum_{b=1}^{B} [\hat{\theta}^*_b - \hat{\theta}^*_B]^2$$

denote the standard bootstrap variance estimator, then

$$\tilde{V}^*_B \leq \hat{V}^*_B.$$

A proof of these assertions can be found in Efron (2014). The estimator $\tilde{V}^*_B$ turns out to be biased upwards if the number of bootstrap samples is too small. Subtracting

$$\frac{N}{B^2} \sum_{b=1}^{B} (\hat{\theta}^*_b - \hat{\theta}^*_B)^2$$

from (6.6) provides a bias reduced estimator (Wager et al., 2014).

The infinitesimal jackknife variance estimator from Theorem 6.2 can be applied to estimate the variance of the bias corrected estimators. For the bias-corrected estimator $\tilde{\theta}_k^*$ one obtains

$$\tilde{V}_k^* = \frac{1}{B^2}\left\{\sum_{n=1}^{N}\left[\sum_{b=1}^{B}(N_{bn}^* - 1)(\tilde{\theta}_{bk}^* - \tilde{\theta}_k^*)\right]^2 - N\sum_{b=1}^{B}(\tilde{\theta}_{bk}^* - \tilde{\theta}_k^*)^2\right\}. \tag{6.8}$$

How well is the infinitesimal jackknife estimator (6.7) doing? Efron (2014) defines three bootstrap confidence intervals, one based on the percentile interval of the estimators from the bootstrap samples, one by $\hat{\theta} \pm 1.96\sqrt{\hat{V}_B^*}$, i.e. using the standard bootstrap estimator of the standard error and one by $\hat{\theta}_B^* \pm 1.96\sqrt{\tilde{V}_B^*}$, i.e. using the infinitesimal jackknife estimator. For the example he considers, the latter has the smallest length. In a comment to Efron's paper, Wang et al. (2014) ran simulations using several model selection techniques like LASSO (Tibshirani, 1996) and best subset selection based on AIC and BIC. They consider linear, Poisson, quantile and non-parametric regression. In all cases, the confidence interval using the infinitesimal jackknife variance was the shortest while providing the required coverage.

6.4 A CASE STUDY

The case study comprises data of patients with advanced prostate carcinoma. It was first analyzed to identify prognostic factors in Byar and Green (1980). Placebo and three dose levels of diethyl stilbestrol were administered in the study, but for the analysis, placebo combined with low dose served as control, the high dose arms as the test treatment. The data were available only with the combined treatment assignment. After removing patients with incomplete data, 475 subjects with complete data remained. Candidate markers were existence of bone metastases, disease stage (3 or 4), performance, history of cardiovascular events, age and weight. For our analysis, age was dichotomized as below or above 65 years and weight as below or above 100 kg.

Let Y_n denote the survival time of subject n and ξ_n an indicator variable equaling 1 if Y_n is observed and zero if censored. T_n denotes the treatment indicator (0 = control, 1 = experimental) and X_{nk} the group indicator (equaling 1 if subject n belongs to subgroup k and zero otherwise). The learning set $\mathcal{L}$ is therefore made up by variables $L_n = (Y_n, \xi_n, \mathbf{X}_n, T_n)$.

We are interested in the marker with the largest impact on the treatment effect. Impact will be measured in terms of the Bayesian information criterion (BIC), a goodness-of-fit measure that is penalized by the number of parameters in the model (Schwartz, 1979):

$$\text{BIC} = K \log(N) - 2 \log(\ell(\hat{\theta}))$$

where $\ell(\hat{\theta})$ denotes the maximum of the likelihood for θ. We are only interested in models with the smallest BIC including the prognostic model, i.e. the model without any treatment by marker interactions, given by (6.9) below. Hence we start with fitting the latter by the Cox model (Cox, 1972)

$$\lambda_0(y) = \lambda(y) \exp\left\{ \alpha_0 + \beta_0 t + \sum_{k=1}^{K} \gamma_k x_k \right\} \quad (6.9)$$

with a BIC equal to g_0. Next we fit the K predictive models

$$\lambda_k(y) = \lambda(y) \exp\left\{ \alpha_k + \beta_k t + \sum_{l=1}^{K} \gamma_l x_l + \delta_k t x_k \right\}. \quad (6.10)$$

Denote the resulting BIC by g_k and define the selection functions u_k, $k = 1, \ldots, K$, by

$$u_k = \begin{cases} 1, & \text{if } g_k = \min(g_0, g_1, \ldots, g_K) \\ 0, & \text{otherwise} \end{cases}. \quad (6.11)$$

In particular if $g_k > g_0$ for all $k = 1, \ldots, K$, no subgroup will be selected.

The treatment by marker interaction estimates are shown in Table 6.1. The model with age group by treatment interaction minimizes BIC among

Table 6.1 Estimates of treatment by subgroup interaction and model fit statistics for prostate cancer data from a proportional hazard model

Subgroup	BIC	$\hat{\delta}_k$	SE	p-value
Age group	3783.4	0.91	0.31	0.0037
Bone metastases	3785.2	−0.74	0.28	0.0074
None	3786.4	—	—	—
CV history	3789.4	0.37	0.22	0.0931
Stage	3789.8	−0.35	0.23	0.1205
Performance	3791.1	0.34	0.33	0.3022
Weight group	3791.8	−0.15	0.23	0.5210

all models considered. This would imply that the test treatment is superior to control in patients of younger rather than old age. Only the inclusion of age group or bone metastases by treatment interaction results in models with smaller BIC than the prognostic model.

Bootstrap samples were drawn from the the prostate cancer data as proposed in Efron (1981). The results of the analysis of 2000 samples are as follows. Table 6.2 shows how often a specific covariate was selected. Despite the fact that age group turned out to be most influential in the learning set it did so in only about 50% of the bootstrap samples The presence of bone metastases was most influential in only 30%, indicating a substantial amount of model uncertainty. The results for the selected covariate age group are summarized in Table 6.3. The between subgroup

Table 6.2 Percentage of covariate selection from 2000 bootstrap samples of the prostate cancer data

Covariate	% selected
Age group	48.55
Bone mets	30.55
CV history	7.45
None	6.40
Stage	3.80
Performance	2.50
Weight group	0.75

Table 6.3 Estimates of treatment effects within and between age groups from 2000 bootstrap samples of the prostate cancer data

Age group	$\hat{\delta}_k$	SE	$\check{\delta}_k^*$	SE	$\tilde{\delta}_k^*$	SE
S0 (< 65 y)	−0.96	0.29	−0.78	0.98	−0.82	0.57
S1 (≥ 65 y)	−0.05	0.12	−0.09	0.12	−0.08	0.15
S1−S0	0.91	0.31	0.69	0.98	0.74	0.50

treatment effect estimators are smaller than the unadjusted ones while the within subgroup estimates are scaled together as best seen in Figure 6.1.

Standard errors for the bias reduced treatment effect estimators are larger than for the non-adjusted estimators as expected accounting for model uncertainty. Replacing the estimator of the selected population with the aggregated estimator from the bootstrap samples reduces the

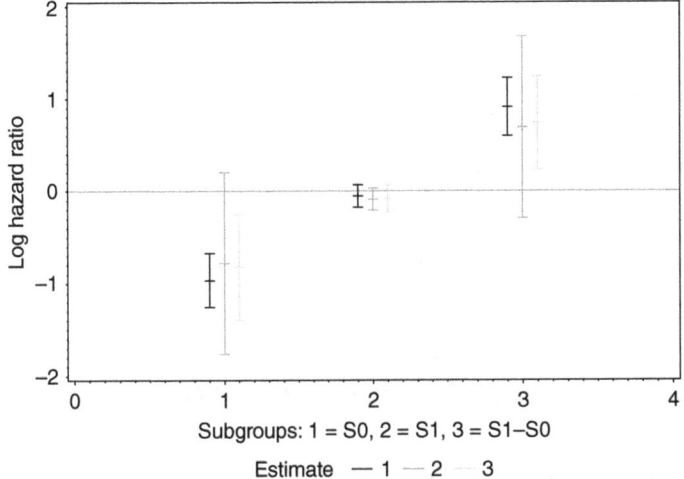

Figure 6.1 Treatment effect estimates in terms of log hazard ratios and standard errors in subgroups and between subgroups for subjects less than 65 or above 65 years of age. Estimates labeled 1 stem from the Cox model on the original data; estimates labeled 2 or 3 are the bias corrected estimates (6.3) and (6.5), respectively.

standard error while the bias is becoming a little larger. It should be noticed that the uncorrected estimator of the hazard ratio between age groups is $\exp(0.91) = 2.48$ while the bias corrected ones are $\exp(0.69) = 1.99$ and $\exp(0.74) = 2.10$, respectively. This corresponds to an optimism of 18% to 25%.

The selection procedure applied above can be regarded as the first step of a forward selection procedure of the interaction effects while the main (prognostic) effects stay in the model. One could extend the procedure to include the full forward selection in the bias adjustment of the estimators.

Another option would be to select all markers whose corresponding BIC is smaller than the BIC of the prognostic model. This would result in selection functions

$$u_k = \begin{cases} 1, & \text{if } g_k < g_0 \\ 0, & \text{otherwise} \end{cases}. \qquad (6.12)$$

6.5 CONCLUDING REMARKS

Since studies are rarely designed under the aspect of subgroup exploration one question will always be whether the sample size is sufficient to reach valid conclusions. For the matter of selection this could mean whether existing subgroups are detectable with good chance, whether the risk to identify artifacts is low, and whether parameters of interest are estimable with acceptable accuracy and precision. Unfortunately there does not seem to be an easy answer to these questions, but simulations of scenarios of interest have to be undertaken to figure out how a method likely performs in terms of relevant characteristics. This can provide a basis to decide whether an analysis is worthwhile to be conducted.

The use of re-sampling methods specifically raises the question about how many samples are needed to achieve accurate and reproducible results. Some hints to this effect are given in Efron and Tibshirani (1993) for the estimation of standard errors and bias and in Efron (2014) for bagged estimators. Generally, estimation of bias requires more re-sampling than variance estimation. Wang et al. (2014) used 4000 samples in their simulations. A pragmatic approach is to increase B until estimates stabilize, which should not cause problems given today's computer power.

SAS code (SAS, 2016) for the case study is provided in the supplementary material of Rosenkranz (2016). The R package `subtee` (Ballarini et al., 2019) implements the bias corrected estimation in a generic way, i.e. for continuous, binary and survival data and produces graphical output.

7

The Predicted Individual Treatment Effect

> At first sight it might seem as though a good model is one that fits the observed data well, ... However, by including a sufficient number of parameters in our model, we may make the fit as close as we please, and indeed by using as many parameters as observations we can make the fit perfect. In so doing, however, we have achieved no reduction in complexity – produced no simple theoretical pattern for the ragged data. Thus simplicity, represented by parsimony of parameters, is also a desirable feature of any model; we do not include parameters that we do not need. (McCullagh and Nelder, 1989)
>
> P McCullagh (1952) and J A Nelder (1924–2010), What is a good model?

7.1 INTRODUCTION

In the previous chapters variable selection was an essential part of subgroup analysis since subgroups had been defined in terms of covariates in a statistical model. Now we turn to an idea where subgroups are defined in terms of the expected advantage of a test treatment over a control treatment given a set of candidate covariates. In this situation variable selection or reduction of the number of variables in the model can be important to increase the accuracy of predictions and estimators and to ease interpretation of the results, but not primarily to characterize subgroups.

In the following we will start from a prediction model that relates treatment benefit with a set of potentially relevant covariates and use this model to predict the differential benefit of the two interventions in a future subject based on the values of his covariates. If the predicted differential benefit favors one treatment over the other by a given amount, the more appropriate treatment would be recommended. This differential benefit is also called the *predicted individual treatment effect* or PITE for short, in contrast to the *average treatment effect* (ATE), which does not consider covariates but overall differences.

To our knowledge, the term PITE was used for the first time in Lamont et al. (2018); however, its definition was proposed earlier in Zhao et al. (2013), Tian et al. (2014), Chen et al. (2017), among others, and essentially builds on the concept of potential outcomes and causal inference (see for example the monograph of Imbens and Rubin (2015)).

After having introduced definitions and notation, we investigate confidence intervals for the PITE under a full data model containing all candidate biomarkers and models after variable selection as obtained from a LASSO fit. The methods are extended to binary and time-to-event data and illustrated in case studies.

7.2 DEFINITION OF THE PITE

Suppose that each subject in a comparative study is randomly assigned to one of two treatments $T = 0$ and $T = 1$, for example a reference and a test treatment. Let $Y(t)$ be the *potential outcome* had the subject been assigned treatment $T = t$. As a consequence, for each subject, only $Y = Y(T) = TY(1) + (1 - T)Y(0)$ can be observed.

Let $\mathbf{X}$ denote the vector of a subject's baseline covariates and let $\mu_t(\mathbf{x})$ be the expected response of a subject with covariates $\mathbf{X} = \mathbf{x}$ assigned treatment $T = t$. The predicted individual treatment effect is the difference between the expected response under treatment 1 and the expected response under treatment 0:

$$D(\mathbf{x}) = \mu_1(\mathbf{x}) - \mu_0(\mathbf{x})$$
$$= E[Y(1)|\mathbf{X} = \mathbf{x}] - E[Y(0)|\mathbf{X} = \mathbf{x}] \quad (7.1)$$

Although the individual differences $Y(1) - Y(0)$ are not known, the expectations $E[Y(0)]$ and $E[Y(1)]$ are estimable if T is independent of $Y(1)$, $Y(0)$ and $\mathbf{X}$. This condition is fulfilled in randomized trials. Let $(y_n, t_n, \mathbf{x}_n)$, $n = 1, \ldots, N$, be the collected data, then $\hat{Y}(t) = \sum_{t_n = t}^{N} y_n / n_t$ with $n_t = \sum_{n=1}^{N} tt_n + (1-t)(1-t_n)$ is an estimator of $E[Y(t)]$, since the missing data are missing completely at random.

Let $\hat{D}(\mathbf{x})$ be an estimator of $D(\mathbf{x})$ and assume that a smaller value of Y indicates a better response, then subjects with $\hat{D}(\mathbf{x}) \leq c$ for some $c < 0$ would potentially be better off under treatment 1.

7.3 CONFIDENCE INTERVALS OF THE PITE

We quote here some results from Ballarini et al. (2018) who investigated how to obtain confidence intervals for the PITE under different model selection approaches. First we consider continuous data and a linear regression model in which the response Y is related to the assigned treatment $T = t$ and K biomarkers $\mathbf{X} = \mathbf{x}$ as

$$Y = \alpha + \beta t + \sum_{k=1}^{K} \gamma_k x_k + t \sum_{k=1}^{K} \delta_k x_k + e \quad (7.2)$$

where e is normally distributed with zero mean and variance σ^2. Under model (7.2) the PITE for a subject with covariates $\mathbf{X} = \mathbf{x}$ is given by

$$D(\mathbf{x}) = \beta + \sum_{k=1}^{K} \delta_k x_k.$$

Let $\theta = (\alpha, \beta, \gamma_1, \ldots, \gamma_k, \delta_1, \ldots, \delta_K)$ and $\mathbf{L} = (0, 1, 0, \ldots, 0, x_1, \ldots, x_K)'$, then the PITE above can be written as linear contrast $D(\mathbf{x}) = \mathbf{L}'\theta$. We consider several approaches to estimate the PITE and to obtain a confidence interval.

7.3.1 MLE for the Full Model

Let $\mathbf{W} = (1, \mathbf{T}, \mathbf{X}, \mathbf{TX})$ denote the design matrix that includes an intercept, treatment, prognostic and predictive effects, and $\hat{\theta}_{\text{MLE}} = (\mathbf{W}'\mathbf{W})^{-1}\mathbf{W}'\mathbf{y}$ the maximum likelihood estimator of θ. Then $\hat{D}(\mathbf{x}) = \mathbf{L}'\hat{\theta}$ and $\text{Var}[\hat{D}(\mathbf{x})] = \sigma^2 \mathbf{L}'(\mathbf{W}'\mathbf{W})^{-1}\mathbf{L}$ where σ^2 can be estimated with

$$S^2 = \frac{1}{N-d}(\mathbf{y}'\mathbf{y} - \hat{\theta}'\mathbf{W}'\mathbf{y}) \qquad (7.3)$$

with $d = 2K + 2$. This allows construction of a $100(1 - \alpha)\%$ confidence interval for $D(\mathbf{x})$ using

$$CI_{\text{MLE}} = [\mathbf{L}'\hat{\theta} \pm t_{N-d, 1-\alpha/2}(S^2 \mathbf{L}'(\mathbf{W}'\mathbf{W})^{-1}\mathbf{L})^{1/2}].$$

7.3.2 MLE Under a Reduced Model

For this method one first selects parameters, e.g. by using the LASSO described below or any other variable selection method, refits the model with the reduced set of parameters, and gets confidence intervals from the reduced model. This procedure is not appropriate since it does not account for selection. It is included for comparison purposes only.

7.3.3 Scheffé Confidence Bounds

To obtain a universally valid post selection confidence interval one can perform simultaneous confidence intervals for the sets of parameters in all possible submodels (Berk et al., 2013). One way to accomplish this is to refer to Scheffé-type confidence bounds (Scheffé, 1953), which provide simultaneous intervals for all possible combinations of parameters. These intervals are given by

$$CI_{\text{Scheffé}} = [\mathbf{L}'\hat{\theta} \pm (dF^\alpha_{d,N-d} S^2 \mathbf{L}'(\mathbf{W}'\mathbf{W})^{-1}\mathbf{L})^{1/2}]$$

where $F^\alpha_{d,N-d}$ denotes the α-quantile of the F-distribution with $(d, N - d)$ degrees of freedom. S^2 can be obtained from (7.3), i.e. from the full model.

7.3.4 LASSO with Post-selection Intervals

To improve estimation accuracy and interpretation in case of many biomarkers, one may perform model selection. The LASSO (Tibshirani, 1996) is a regularization technique for simultaneous estimation and variable selection. LASSO estimates are obtained from

$$\hat{\theta}_{\text{LASSO}} = \operatorname{argmin}\left\{\frac{1}{N}\|\mathbf{y} - \mathbf{W}'\theta\|_2^2 + \lambda\|\theta\|_1\right\} \quad (7.4)$$

where $\|.\|_p$ denotes the L^p-norm and $\lambda \geq 0$ is a regularization parameter.

The LASSO starts with model (7.2) but provides automatic model selection through shrinkage of the estimates of the model parameters to the extent that some may vanish. This leads to a set of active predictors $\mathcal{P} = \{i; \theta_i \neq 0\}$. Recent work in selective inference (Taylor and Tibshirani, 2017) have provided new tools for developing confidence intervals for LASSO estimates. These methods allow to construct confidence intervals for the PITE from the LASSO conditional on the selected model $\mathcal{P}$. However, when conditioning on the selected model, the target of inference changes (Berk et al., 2013). Instead of considering the full model one is now making inferences towards a potentially reduced model. The confidence intervals are designed such that

$$P_{\theta_\mathcal{P}}[\mathbf{L}'_\mathcal{P}\theta_\mathcal{P} \in CI_{\text{LASSO}}|\mathcal{P}] = 1 - \alpha$$

where $\mathbf{L}_\mathcal{P}$ and $\theta_\mathcal{P}$ denote the subvectors of $\mathcal{L}$ and θ corresponding to the selected parameters in $\mathcal{P}$.

When implementing the LASSO, covariates should be standardized such that they have the same variance and are equally penalized. However, when performing the LASSO with interactions, the variables should first be standardized before forming the interactions with treatments. For more details see Ballarini et al. (2018).

7.3.5 Randomized LASSO

The disadvantage of selective inference is that it may result in very wide confidence intervals (Kivaranovic and Leeb, 2018). To obtain narrower confidence intervals, a randomized response can be used in the LASSO (Tian and Taylor, 2018). The original response Y is replaced by $Y^* = Y + U$ for a random U and the LASSO is applied to the new outcome. We consider $U \sim N(0, q\sigma^2)$ for some $q > 0$. However, the gain comes at the cost of a reduced quality of model selection because of the additional noise.

7.3.6 Simulation Study

The methods described above are applied to simulated datasets to evaluate their statistical properties, in particular the bias and the mean squared error (MSE) and the coverage of the confidence interval.

Bias and MSE are defined as $E[E[\hat{D}(\mathbf{X}) - D(\mathbf{X})]]$ and $E[E[(\hat{D}(\mathbf{X}) - D(\mathbf{X}))^2]]$, respectively. The inner expectation is with respect to $\mathbf{X}$, the covariate of a future subject, and the outer expectation with respect to the learning dataset on which the model is fit.

The selective inference procedure aims to control the conditional coverage probability

$P[\hat{D}_l(\mathbf{x}) < D_{\mathcal{P}}(\mathbf{x}) < \hat{D}_u(\mathbf{x})|\mathcal{P}]$ for all fixed covariate vectors $\mathbf{x}$, where $D_{\mathcal{P}}(\mathbf{x})$ is the true value of the PITE under the selected model $\mathcal{P}$, which may differ for each estimation method. In the results we report the overall expected coverage probability $P[\hat{D}_l(\mathbf{X}) < D_{\mathcal{P}}(\mathbf{X}) < \hat{D}_u(\mathbf{X})]$ where we average over the distribution of $\mathbf{X}$ and the distribution of the learning dataset.

We use sample sizes $N = 40, 100, 220,$ and 350 with an allocation ratio of one. Data are generated as $Y_n = \mu_n + e_n$ with $e_n \sim N(0, 1)$. The mean depends on the baseline covariates through

$$\mu_n = \alpha + \beta t_n + \gamma_1 x_{1n} + \gamma_2 x_{2n} + \delta_1 x_{1n} t_n + \delta_2 x_{2n} t_n$$

where $t_n \in \{-1, 1\}$ is the treatment variable. The two covariates are simulated from distributions with zero mean and unit variance, namely a binary variable attaining -1 and 1 with equal probability and the other variable being uniformly distributed on $[-\sqrt{3}, \sqrt{3}]$. In addition, eight normally distributed variables with mean zero and unit variance are simulated, resulting in $K = 10$, which is not used to simulated data but for the analysis. Two scenarios are run: a null model with $\alpha = \beta = \gamma_1 = \gamma_2 = \delta_1 = \delta_2 = 0$ and a predictive model with $\alpha = \beta = \gamma_1 = \delta_1 = 0.12$ and $\gamma_2 = \delta_2 = 0.29$. Simulation results can be summarized as follows:

- While the MLE based on the full model provides unbiased estimates, the MSE is larger than for the other methods.

- Performing model selection with the LASSO provides biased estimates but with a gain in MSE.
- The confidence intervals for the LASSO can become quite wide, particularly when the sample size is small. The randomized LASSO is a superior alternative.
- The reduced model provides the narrowest confidence intervals, but are invalid because they do not have the required coverage.
- The Scheffé bounds in the reduced model are wide and their coverage is way above what is requested.

The results for the confidence intervals are depicted in Figure 7.1. For detailed data on bias and MSE we refer to table 2 of Ballarini et al. (2018). Further simulations contained in the supplements of this paper show that when the number of biomarkers is substantially larger the shrinkage methods offer a clear advantage in the PITE estimation. In a completely exploratory setting with very large numbers of biomarkers and small sample size the uncertainty of the model selection may lead to wide confidence intervals that may be uninformative. Simulation results for correlated biomarkers are similar to those in the independent case.

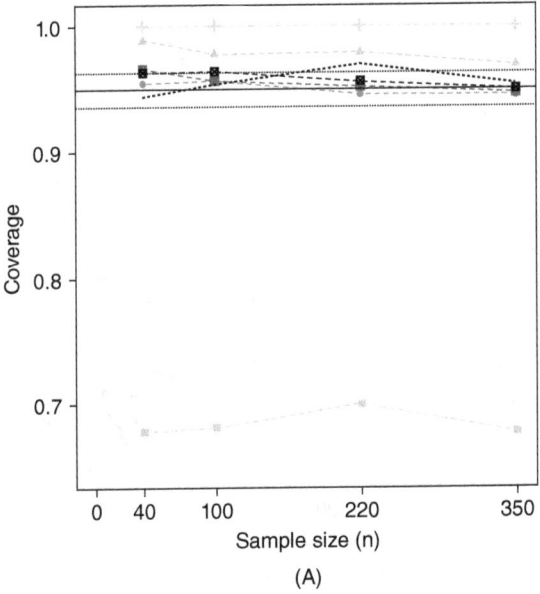

Figure 7.1 Average coverage of the confidence intervals for the PITE in (A) the null case and (B) the predicted case. The solid line at 95% indicates the target coverage and the bands around them indicate ±1.96 standard error of the simulations. ATE denotes the average treatment effect obtained from model (7.2) without interactions. rLASSO-1 and rLASSO-2 have $q = 0.2$ and $q = 0.8$, respectively (see legend on next page).

7.3.7 Extension to Other Endpoints

There are several options to extend the PITE concept to binary and survival data. We choose log odds ratios for the former and log hazard ratios for the latter as a metric for treatment effects, mainly

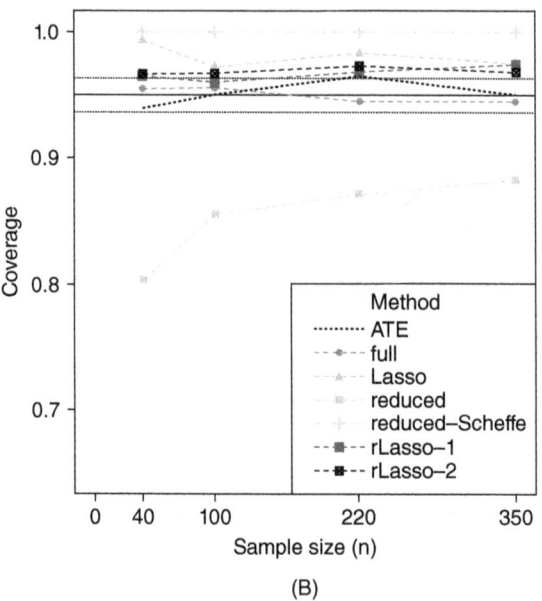

(B)

Figure 7.1 (*Continued*)

because it does not change the mathematical expression of the PITE when data are modeled by a logistic regression or proportional hazards model.

For example for a binary endpoint, let $\pi(\mathbf{x}, t) = E(Y|\mathbf{x}, t] = P[Y = 1|\mathbf{x}, t]$ and $\text{logit}(p) = \log(p/(1-p))$ for $0 < p < 1$. Then

$$\text{logit}(\pi(\mathbf{x}, t)) = \alpha + \beta t + \sum_{k=1}^{K} \gamma_k x_k + t \sum_{k=1}^{K} \delta_k x_k$$

and

$$D(\mathbf{x}) = \text{logit}(\pi(\mathbf{x}, 1)) - \text{logit}(\pi(\mathbf{x}, 0))$$
$$= \beta + \sum_{k=1}^{K} \delta_k x_k.$$

Similarly, for the proportional hazards model

$$\lambda(y, \mathbf{x}, t) = \lambda_0(y) \exp\left\{\beta t + \sum_{k=1}^{K} \gamma_k x_k + t \sum_{k=1}^{K} \delta_k x_k\right\} \quad (7.5)$$

one obtains

$$D(\mathbf{x}) = \log \lambda(y, \mathbf{x}, 1) - \log \lambda(y, \mathbf{x}, 0)$$
$$= \beta + \sum_{k=1}^{K} \delta_k x_k.$$

In general, the same trends as for normal data can be observed for time-to-event data. Confidence intervals derived from the selected inference framework attain the desired coverage for the PITE while Wald confidence intervals under the reduced model fail to do so. The last example is a re-analysis of a safety study where the emphasis is not on variable selection but on correct subgroup identification.

7.4 CASE STUDIES

In the following we present two illustrations of variable selection for a PITE for continuous normal data and time-to-event data using the LASSO or the randomized LASSO. The survival example is also considered under forward selection and a confidence interval obtained by bootstrapping to see whether the results differ.

7.4.1 An Alzheimer Dataset

This dataset referenced in Schnell et al. (2016) is taken from the clinical development of an Alzheimer's drug undertaken by AbbVie. Unfortunately, no reference is provided for the publication of the results of the corresponding trial. There were 41 subjects treated, 25 receiving placebo ($t = 0$) and 16 receiving test treatment ($t = 1$). Four candidate biomarkers were recorded at baseline: disease severity at study entry (with high values indicating severe cognitive impairment), age, sex, and presence or absence of a genetic marker potentially related to Alzheimer's disease. The response of interest is change in disease severity from baseline to end of study where a negative change refers to improvement. We also added six standard normal variables without any effect on response.

LASSO and randomized LASSO were fit using the glmnet package (Friedman et al., 2010) with regularization parameter $\lambda = 0.1654$. For the randomized LASSO the noise added corresponds to $q = 0.2$. For further details see Ballarini et al. (2018). The parameter estimates and confidence intervals are presented in Figure 7.2A. The variables sex and age were selected when analyzing the data with LASSO and randomized LASSO. The former, however, also selected the interactions of three of the non-predictive variables and produced very wide intervals. The PITE for selected combinations of age and sex is shown in Figure 7.2B.

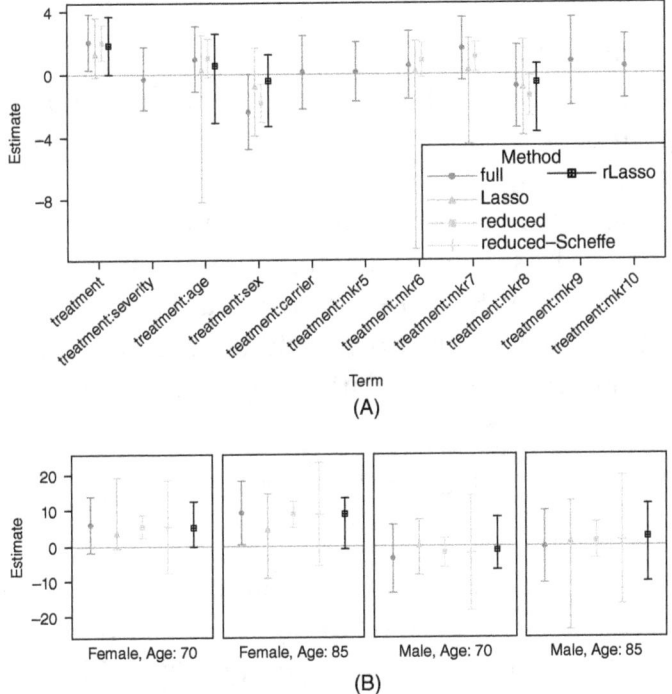

Figure 7.2 Estimates and confidence intervals for model parameters (A) and four selected subjects (B) for the Alzheimer dataset.

The shortest confidence intervals stem from the reduced model, but they are invalid, as already pointed out. Scheffé intervals are widest, as expected, while the intervals from the full model and the randomized LASSO are similar.

7.4.2 The Prostate Cancer Study Again

We fit again a proportional hazards model with treatment by covariate interaction terms (7.5) to the prostate cancer data of Byar and Green (1980) introduced in Chapter 6. Note that this time we include the variables age and weight directly into the model without dichotomizing them as done previously.

As shown in the previous section, $D(\mathbf{x})$ can be estimated as a linear combination of the partial maximum likelihood estimates $\hat{\beta}$ and $\hat{\delta}_k$. The predicted benefit of a future individual with covariates $\mathbf{x}_0$ from the same population is then given by

$$\hat{D}(\mathbf{x}_0) = \hat{\beta} + \sum_{k=1}^{K} \hat{\delta}_k x_{0k}. \qquad (7.6)$$

Estimates of the standard deviation of $\hat{D}(\mathbf{x}_0)$ and confidence intervals for $D(\mathbf{x}_0)$ can be obtained in the usual way (Wald statistics or profile likelihood).

To decide whether all six covariates in the prostate cancer data are necessary to predict a treatment effect, we use two methods: the LASSO and forward selection. Note that main effects and interaction effects are handled independently of each other such that an interaction effect can be added to the model even if the corresponding main effect is not selected. For the calculations we have standardized all independent variables such that they are all on the same scale.

The LASSO is fitted with $\lambda = 0.0454$, following recommendations in Lee et al. (2016). The interactions that stay in the model are the ones between treatment and age or bone metastases. The estimated model parameters and their confidence intervals shown in Figure 7.3. Figure 7.4 shows

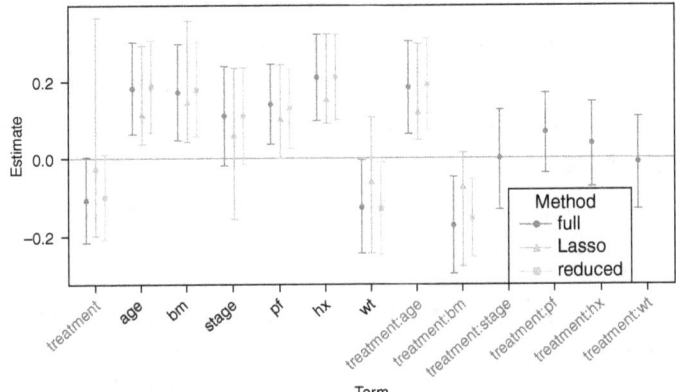

Figure 7.3 Parameter estimates and confidence intervals for the prostate cancer study. Full refers to a Cox model including all variables, and reduced to a Cox model including only the variables selected by the LASSO.

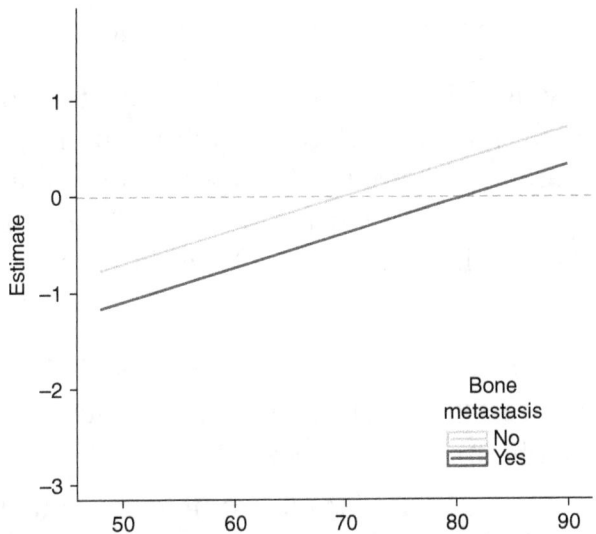

Figure 7.4 PITE for combinations of levels of age and bone metastases for the prostate cancer study.

the PITE and confidence intervals when using the LASSO for combinations of levels of the selected covariates. For patients with bone metastases, treatment 1 would still be beneficial at a higher age.

The alternative analysis (forward selection) is done as follows:

1. Start with the null model, i.e. all parameters are set to zero.
2. Compute the score statistic for every effect not in the model.
3. If the largest score statistics is significant at a pre-set entry level, the effect is added to the model
4. Repeat steps 2 and 3 until none of the effects not in the model meets the entry criterion.

Applying this algorithm to the prostate cancer data picks all main effects as well as the interactions between treatment and age or bone metastasis, as in the analysis using the LASSO. To obtain a confidence interval for $D(\mathbf{x}_0)$ one can proceed as follows:

1. For $b = 1, \ldots, B$, fit the Cox model (7.5) with forward selection to bootstrap sample $\mathcal{L}_b^*$ from $\mathcal{L}$ to obtain $\hat{D}_b^*(\mathbf{x}_0) = \hat{D}(\mathbf{x}_0, \mathcal{L}_b^*)$.
2. For a $100(1 - 2\alpha)\%$ confidence interval for $D(\mathbf{x}_0)$ take the 100αth upper and lower percentile of the distribution of $\{\hat{D}_1^*(\mathbf{x}_0), \ldots, \hat{D}_B^*(\mathbf{x}_0)\}$.

Figure 7.5 shows the PITE for four different individuals characterized by an age of 60 or 80 and the presence or absence of bone metastases. The confidence intervals after model selection (marked as Y) are too short since they do not account for variable selection. The bootstrap derived intervals are wider than those from the full model indicating that the lower variability of the sparser model is more than compensated by the uncertainty of selecting the right variables. From a medical point of view this analysis shows that younger subjects with bone metastases benefit most from test treatment while test treatment may be harmful to older patients without bone metastases. This result is in agreement with the LASSO analysis as well.

7.4.3 Renal Safety of Contrast Media

Contrast-induced nephropathy (CIN) is a serious complication of diagnostic and interventional procedures. In McCullough et al. (2006) the risk of nephrotoxicity was compared under two contrast media, isosmolar iodixanol (IOCM) and a low-osmolar medium (LOCM). Furthermore the authors set out to identify predictors of contrast induced nephropathy. An individual patient data meta analysis including 2727 patients from 16 double-blind, randomized, controlled trials with stratification according to chronic kidney disease (CKD) and diabetes mellitus (DM) was performed. Endpoints were increase in serum creatinine (Cr)

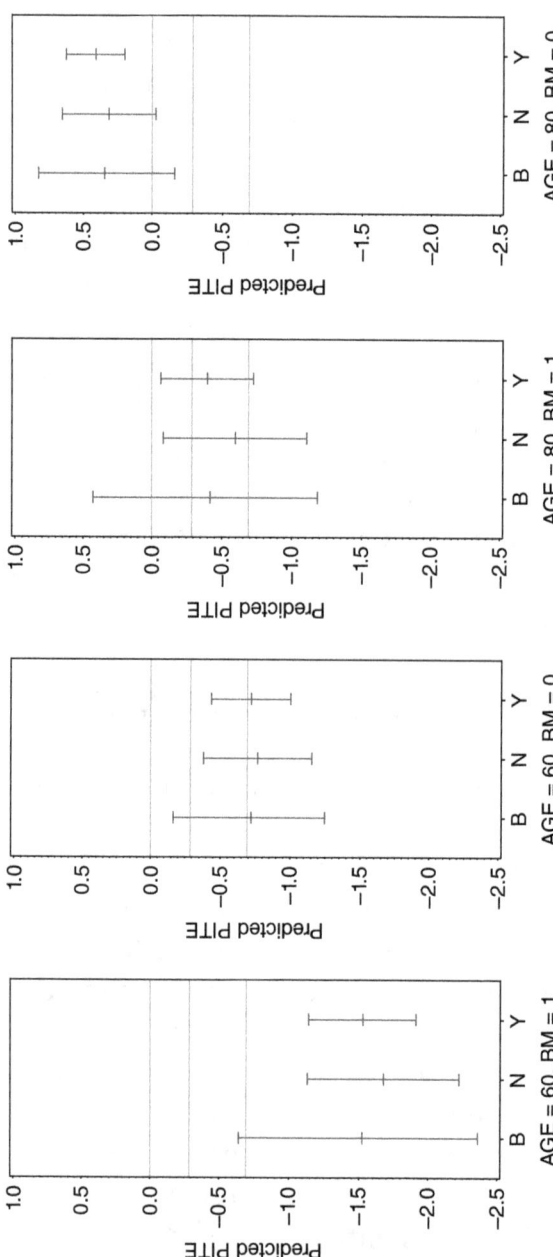

Figure 7.5 PITEs and 90% confidence intervals for different subject characteristics. N stands for no, Y for forward selection without adjustment and B for forward selection with intervals derived from 1000 bootstrap samples. The three horizontal lines correspond to no, a 25%, or a 50% hazard reduction of test versus control.

and incidence of post procedural contrast-induced nephropathy, defined as a rise in creatinine by more than $0.5\,\mathrm{mg\,dl^{-1}}$. The CIN rates by subgroups are shown in Table 7.1. Although the data stem from 16 randomized trials, only summary data are reported in the paper by McCullough et al. (2006). The authors conclude that "Patient-related predictors of CIN were found to be CKD and CKD + DM, but not DM alone." These predictors correspond to the subgroups with a significant *p*-value for a within-subgroup comparison in Table 7.1.

We will now re-analyze the CIN data using the PITE methodology as in Rosenkranz (2017). For our analysis we fitted a saturated logistic model to the data. Let X_1, X_2 denote the indicator variables for CKD and DM, respectively, let T denote the treatment indicator with $T = 0$ coding for IOCM and $T = 1$ for LOCM. Let $p(t, \mathbf{x})$ be the probability of CIN in a patient with covariates $\mathbf{X} = \mathbf{x}$ treated with $T = t$. Then the probability $p(t, \mathbf{x})$ that a subject suffers from CIN under treatment t given covariates $\mathbf{x}$ can be modeled as

$$\mathrm{logit}(p(t, \mathbf{x})) = \alpha + \beta t + \gamma_1 x_1 + \gamma_2 x_2 + \gamma_3 x_1 x_2 \\ + t(\delta_1 x_1 + \delta_2 x_2 + \delta_3 x_1 x_2). \quad (7.7)$$

The prognostic effects describe the dependence of the response under treatment $T = 0$ while the predictive effects account for the additional impact of the covariates under $T = 1$.

Table 7.1 Number of patients with CIN over total number of patients by patient subgroups and contrast media from McCullough et al. (2006). CI = confidence interval, CKD = chronic kidney disease, DM = diabetes mellitus, IOCM = isomolar contrast media, LOCM = low-osmolar contrast media, OR = odds ratio. p-values are from Fisher's exact test

Population	IOCM	LOCM	OR (95% CI)	p-value
All	19/1382	47/1340	0.38 (0.22–0.66)	<0.001
CKD = Y	10/362	31/371	0.31 (0.15–0.65)	0.001
CKD = N	9/1020	16/969	0.53 (0.23–1.21)	0.160
CKD = Y, DM = Y	4/115	18/116	0.20 (0.06–0.65)	0.003
CKD = Y, DM = N	6/247	13/255	0.46 (0.17–1.24)	0.16
CKD = N, DM = Y	1/178	3/158	0.29 (0.03–2.84)	0.35
CKD = N, DM = N	8/842	13/811	0.59 (0.24–1.43)	0.28

We fitted model (7.7) to the learning data set in Table 7.1 and obtained the results in Table 7.2. The odds ratios and confidence intervals are identical to those in table 4 of McCullough et al. (2006); however, the *p*-values differ since we took the results of the asymptotic tests from the logistic model rather than from Fisher's exact test as was done in the paper. Nevertheless, the results are practically identical since the corresponding comparisons result in either very small or large *p*-values. Note that the comparison of patients with and without diabetes was not presented in McCullough et al. (2006), though the authors explicitly excluded DM from being predictive on its own.

Tables 7.1 and 7.2 show the problems of deciding on subgroup effects based on tests within subgroups. The effect of medium is significant on the 5% level for subjects with CKD regardless of the DM status and vice versa, but not significant for subjects with CKD in the absence of DM nor in subjects with DM in the absence of CKD.

The PITE corresponding to model (7.7) is given by the log odds ratio

$$D(\mathbf{x}) = \text{logit}\{p(1,\mathbf{x})\} - \text{logit}\{p(0,\mathbf{x})\}$$
$$= \beta + \delta_1 x_1 + \delta_2 x_2 + \delta_3 x_1 x_2.$$

Note that the PITE does not depend on prognostic effects and that

$$\exp\{D(\mathbf{x})\} = \frac{p(1,\mathbf{x})[1 - p(0,\mathbf{x})]}{[1 - p(1,\mathbf{x})]p(0,\mathbf{x})} = \text{OR}(\mathbf{x})$$

Table 7.2 Odds ratios of the risk of CIN under contrast medium 1 relative to medium O. Odds ratios and confidence intervals are identical to those in table 4 of McCullough et al. (2006). p-values differ from those of Fisher's exact test that are presented in the paper

Subgroup	Events/patients	OR (95% CI)	p-value
All	66/2722	0.38 (0.22–0.66)	0.0005
CKD = Y	41/733	0.31 (0.15–0.65)	0.0017
CKD = N	25/1989	0.53 (0.23–1.21)	0.1301
DM = Y	26/567	0.29 (0.08–0.56)	0.0019
DM = N	40/2155	0.52 (0.27–1.00)	0.0511
CKD = Y, DM = Y	22/231	0.20 (0.06–0.60)	0.0043
CKD = Y, DM = N	19/502	0.46 (0.17–1.24)	0.1254
CKD = N, DM = Y	4/336	0.29 (0.03–2.84)	0.2885
CKD = N, DM = N	21/1653	0.59 (0.24–1.43)	0.2414

is the odds ratio of the probability to experience CIN under medium 1 relative to medium 0 for a subject with covariates $\mathbf{x}$. Let $\hat{\beta}$ and $\hat{\delta}_i$ be the maximum likelihood (ML) estimators of β and δ_i, respectively, then

$$\hat{D}(\mathbf{x}) = \hat{\beta} + \hat{\delta}_1 x_1 + \hat{\delta}_2 x_2 + \hat{\delta}_3 x_1 x_2$$

is the ML estimator of $D(\mathbf{x})$. A predictor for the most appropriate treatment of a future patient with covariates $\mathbf{x}_0$ is therefore

$$\hat{\varphi}_D(\mathbf{x}_0, c) = \begin{cases} 1, & \text{if } \hat{D}(\mathbf{x}_0) \leq c \\ 0, & \text{otherwise} \end{cases}.$$

For the CIN data we may decide that medium 1 should be preferred over medium 0 when the observed reduction of CIN risk is 50% or more. In other words, medium 0 should not be given to subjects when the CIN risk over medium 1 more than doubles relative to medium 1. A predictor for the best treatment is therefore given by $\hat{\varphi}_D(\mathbf{x}_0, \log(0.5))$. This rule should be reasonable since the overall CIN risks are 3.5% for medium 0 and 1.4% for medium 1. According to this decision rule, all subjects with DM or CKD or both should be given contrast medium 1.

The decision rule based on the PITE depends solely on the point estimates of the odds ratios. To obtain a measure of reliability one can use the bootstrap again to check how many samples drawn from the learning data would result in the same decision. Here we use the parametric bootstrap that re-samples from the parameter estimates of a known distribution rather than from the empirical distribution function since we do not know the original data but only summary statistics.

In our case let $N(t, \mathbf{x})$ be the number of subjects with $T = t$ and $\mathbf{X} = \mathbf{x}$ in the learning set and let $n(t, \mathbf{x})$ be the number of those subjects with CIN. For $b = 1, \ldots, B$, we draw new random numbers $n_b^*(t, \mathbf{x})$ from a binomial distribution with parameters $n(t, \mathbf{x})/N(t, \mathbf{x})$ and $N(t, \mathbf{x})$ and obtain the corresponding PITE estimates $\hat{D}_b^*(\mathbf{x})$. Then

$$\hat{P}_B^*(\mathbf{x}, c) = \frac{1}{B} \sum_{b=1}^{B} \hat{\varphi}_{D_b^*}(\mathbf{x}, c) \qquad (7.8)$$

is an estimator of the probability that a subject with covariates $\mathbf{x}$ will be assigned medium 1 again if the learning dataset was replicated. The results of the re-analysis are shown in Table 7.3.

Table 7.3 Predicted odds ratio and proportions of $B = 1000$ bootstrap samples leading to a preference of contrast medium 1 for a future subject with covariates $\mathbf{x}_0$

x_{01}	x_{02}	$\widehat{OR}(\mathbf{x}_0)$	$\hat{\varphi}_D(\mathbf{x}_0, \log(0.5))$	$\hat{P}^*(\mathbf{x}_0, \log(0.5))$
1	1	0.20	1	0.977
1	0	0.46	1	0.546
0	1	0.29	1	0.623
0	0	0.59	0	0.342

According to the selection criterion, the subgroups of patients with CDK or DM or both are better off with medium 1 while medium 0 is acceptable for the other subjects. The replicability of a decision in favor of medium 1 is above 50% up to almost 98% for the first three subgroups.

7.5 CONCLUDING REMARKS

The concept of the predicted individual treatment effect is investigating heterogeneity of treatment effects without identifying subgroups explicitly. It rather builds on the direct relationship between an outcome and covariates and uses variable selection primarily to reduce the variability or shorten the confidence intervals of the PITE. The approach allows including covariates directly in the model without having to dichotomize continuous variables in order to obtain subgroups. On the other hand, as pointed out in Breiman (2001), one relies heavily on the appropriateness of the chosen model to describe the outcome–covariate relationship, a question which is often difficult to investigate.

Generally, confidence intervals for the PITE after model selection can be obtained by bootstrapping, i.e, by repeating the selection process on a series of bootstrap samples and using the percentile method to obtain the limits of the interval as shown for one of the examples. There are some theoretical results available on post-selection inference (Berk et al., 2013; Bachoc et al., 2019), which is an area of active research. If variable selection is performed by the LASSO or variants thereof, exact confidence limits exist if the interval is calculated on the condition that a specific model was selected (Hastie et al., 2015; Lee et al., 2016; Taylor and Tibshirani, 2017), which may be unacceptably wide (Kivaranovic and Leeb, 2018) and which may be correctable by introducing randomized response (Tian and Taylor, 2018). Although there are still open questions, tremendous progress has been made.

The proposed intervals are confidence intervals for the PITE, rather than prediction intervals for the subject-level difference in the potential outcomes under two treatments. Developing such prediction intervals requires an estimate of the subject-level correlation of potential outcomes. Since no study participants are observed under both conditions in parallel study designs, there is no empirical information on this dependence. We propose an approach to prediction in the next chapter.

Exploratory Subgroup Analyses in Clinical Research,
First Edition. Gerd Rosenkranz.
© 2020 John Wiley & Sons Ltd. Published 2020 by John Wiley & Sons Ltd.
Companion website: www.wiley.com/go/rosenkranz/exploratory

8

Prediction models

Upon my return, I started reading the Annals of Statistics, the flagship journal of theoretical statistics, and was bemused. Every article started with "Assume that the data are generated by the following model: ..." followed by mathematics exploring inference, hypothesis testing and asymptotics... Statisticians in applied research consider data modeling as the template for statistical analysis: Faced with an applied problem, think of a data model. This enterprise has at its heart the belief that a statistician, by imagination and by looking at the data, can invent a reasonably good parametric class of models for a complex mechanism devised by nature. (Breiman, 2001)

Leo Breiman (1928–2005)—Statistical Modeling: The Two Cultures

8.1 INTRODUCTION

So far the discussion has focused on the estimation of parameters or contrasts thereof (like the PITE) in a supposed data model. Of interest were also the corresponding measures of statistical accuracy like standard errors, biases of estimators and confidence intervals for parameters of the assumed model. The operating characteristics of these statistics were determined by simulation and compared to the true model, which of course is known in simulations. However, measures of accuracy like bias or MSE cannot be derived from the data alone without knowing the true values of model parameters.

Prediction aims to take the model built from a learning dataset to predict the outcome of a future observation. In the context of this book it means that, based on a set of biomarkers or covariates of a future individual, we would like to predict the effect of a treatment. Prediction error measures how well a model allows the prediction of the response of a future observation. This measure of accuracy can be obtained from the data as soon as a predictor has been chosen. As we show, the prediction error accounts for the variability of the data in the learning set and the appropriateness of the predictor.

In this chapter we first recall the definitions of predictor and prediction error and how to estimate the latter. Then we apply the concept to the predictive individual treatment effect in order to predict the difference of the effect that one treatment may have over a control in a future individual. As we will see, the solution to this problem remains incomplete mainly because the potential outcomes are not observable for both treatments but only for one.

8.2 PREDICTION ERROR

Let $\mathcal{L} = \{(y_n, \mathbf{x}_n, t_n)\}$ denote a learning set made up by random draws $(Y, \mathbf{X}, T)$ where Y denotes the response to a treatment T in an individual characterized by covariates $\mathbf{X}$. We assume that covariates $\mathbf{X}$ and treatment assignment T are independent, or formally

$$P(Y, \mathbf{X}, T) = P(Y|\mathbf{X}, T)P(\mathbf{X})P(T).$$

From $\mathcal{L}$ a predictor $\eta(\mathbf{x}, t, \mathcal{L})$ is devised that assigns a predicted outcome y to covariates $\mathbf{X} = \mathbf{x}$ and treatment $T = t$ given $\mathcal{L}$. Prediction error is a quantity that measures how well a predictor derived from a learning dataset predicts the response of a future individual.

In regression models for continuous data, prediction error refers to the expected squared difference (or the squared-error loss) between a future response Y_0 for $(\mathbf{X}_0, T_0)$ and its prediction for a given learning set $\mathcal{L}$:

$$\mathrm{PE}(\mathcal{L}) = E_P[\{Y_0 - \eta(\mathbf{X}_0, T_0, \mathcal{L})\}^2]. \quad (8.1)$$

The expectation refers to repeated sampling from the distribution $P(Y, \mathbf{X}, T)$ for fixed $\mathcal{L}$. For classification problems where Y takes on one of several numbers representing unordered classes like success or failure, the prediction error is commonly defined as the probability of an incorrect classification:

$$\text{PE}(\mathcal{L}) = P[Y_0 \neq \eta(\mathbf{X}_0, T_0, \mathcal{L})]. \quad (8.2)$$

The prediction error accounts for the *model error* (ME), i.e. the difference between the prediction model and the true data model, and the *random error* of the data Y. To see this assume $Y = \mu(\mathbf{X}, T) + e$ where $E[e] = 0$, $E[e^2] = \sigma^2$ and e is independent of $\mathbf{X}$ and T. Then for a predictor $\eta(\mathbf{x}, t, \mathcal{L})$

$$\text{PE}(\mathcal{L}) = E[\{\mu(\mathbf{X}_0, T_0) + e - \eta(\mathbf{X}_0, T_0, \mathcal{L})\}^2]$$
$$= \sigma^2 + E[\{\mu(\mathbf{X}_0, T_0) - \eta(\mathbf{X}_0, T_0, \mathcal{L})\}^2]$$
$$= \sigma^2 + \text{ME}(\mathcal{L}).$$

The model error can be estimated by subtracting an estimator of the random error from an estimator of the prediction error. A naive estimator of the prediction error (8.1) is

$$\widehat{\text{PE}}(\mathcal{L}) = \frac{1}{N} \sum_{n=1}^{N} (y_n - \eta(\mathbf{x}_n, t_n, \mathcal{L}))^2. \quad (8.3)$$

This estimator, called the *apparent error*, will likely be too optimistic since it uses the learning dataset from which the predictor was built to assess model accuracy.

In order to get a more realistic estimate of prediction error one would like to have a test sample that is independent of the learning sample. Ideally that would come in from new data from the same population that produced the learning set. One would then run the data from the test set through the predictor built from the learning set and assess the prediction accuracy.

When additional data are not available, which is often the case, cross-validation uses parts of the data to build the predictor and a different part to test it (Stone, 1974). Alternatively, several bootstrap methods have been developed (Efron, 1983; Efron and Tibshirani, 1997). Breiman and Spector (1992) studied submodel selection in linear regression and found bootstrap to perform well in model selection and estimation of the model error. In a simulation study investigating split-sample, cross-validation, and bootstrapping in providing a more accurate estimate of prediction error with a logistic regression model, the regular bootstrap performed among the best (Steyerberg et al., 2001). We will therefore focus on this method in the following.

For the regular bootstrap procedure, the model is estimated in a bootstrap sample and evaluated in the bootstrap sample and the original sample. The difference between the prediction errors is an estimate of the *optimism* in the apparent error. This difference is averaged over a series of bootstrap samples to obtain a stable estimate of the optimism.

Let $\mathcal{L}_b^* = \{(y_{bn}^*, \mathbf{x}_{bn}^*, t_{bn}^*)\}$ be a bootstrap sample from $\mathcal{L}$ and $\eta(\mathbf{x}, t, \mathcal{L}_b^*)$ a predictor obtained from fitting the sample $\mathcal{L}_b^*$. The apparent error for the fit to the bth bootstrap sample is

$$\widehat{PE}(\mathcal{L}_b^*) = \frac{1}{N} \sum_{n=1}^{N} (y_{bn}^* - \eta(\mathbf{x}_{bn}^*, t_{bn}^*, \mathcal{L}_b^*))^2. \quad (8.4)$$

Using the original sample $\mathcal{L}$ as a test sample, the predictive error estimate is

$$\widehat{PE}(\mathcal{L}, \mathcal{L}_b^*) = \frac{1}{N} \sum_{n=1}^{N} (y_n - \eta(\mathbf{x}_n, t_n, \mathcal{L}_b^*))^2. \quad (8.5)$$

An estimator of the optimism of the apparent error (8.3) is then

$$\widehat{OPE}(\mathcal{L}) = \frac{1}{B} \sum_{b=1}^{B} (\widehat{PE}(\mathcal{L}, \mathcal{L}_b^*) - \widehat{PE}(\mathcal{L}_b^*)). \quad (8.6)$$

A more realistic estimator of prediction error is therefore $\widehat{PE}^*(\mathcal{L}) = \widehat{PE}(\mathcal{L}) + \widehat{OPE}(\mathcal{L})$.

8.3 MODEL SELECTION OR AVERAGING

So far we have described how to obtain an estimator of the prediction error of a predictor based on a given set of candidate covariates. In many cases, the prediction error can be reduced by decreasing the number of variables in the prediction model even if the true predictor contains many non-zero coefficients (Breiman and Spector, 1992).

Many classical variable selection models like forward selection or backward elimination proceed in a sequential way producing a sequence of subsets $\zeta_0, \ldots, \zeta_K$, where ζ_k denotes the indices of the k variables in the model. The predictor based on the subset ζ is denoted by $\eta(\mathbf{x}, t, \mathcal{L}, \zeta)$ and the corresponding prediction error is

$$\text{PE}(\mathcal{L}, \zeta) = E_P[\{Y_0 - \eta(\mathbf{X}_0, T_0, \mathcal{L}, \zeta)\}^2]. \quad (8.7)$$

The idea is to estimate the prediction error for $\zeta_1, \ldots, \zeta_K$ using the regular bootstrap and to choose a submodel ζ_k with

$$\widehat{\text{PE}}(\mathcal{L}, \zeta_k) = \min_{1 \leq k' \leq K} \widehat{\text{PE}}(\mathcal{L}, \zeta_{k'}).$$

Is the selected submodel ζ_k the best predictor in terms of prediction error? Let $\eta(\mathbf{x}, t, \mathcal{L}, \zeta_1), \ldots, \eta(\mathbf{x}, t, \mathcal{L}, \zeta_K)$ be the predictors obtained from the learning set $\mathcal{L}$ and $\eta(\mathbf{x}, t, \mathcal{L}_b^*, \zeta_{1b}^*), \ldots, \eta(\mathbf{x}, t, \mathcal{L}_b^*, \zeta_{Kb}^*)$ the predictors obtained from a bootstrap sample $\mathcal{L}_b^*$. The latter will be averaged to give the sequence of model-averaged predictors

$$\eta_k^*(\mathbf{x}, t, \mathcal{L}) = \frac{1}{B} \sum_{b=1}^{B} \eta(\mathbf{x}, t, \mathcal{L}_b^*, \zeta_{kb}^*), \quad k = 1, \ldots, K.$$

It turns out that for small K, the prediction error of the averaged estimators tends to be smaller than for the original ones; however, there is a point from which this relationship reverses. The explanation is that instability of the predictor increases as the number of variables in the predictor decreases, in which case averaging provides more accurate predictors (Breiman, 1996).

The advantage of a more accurate predictor has a prize. The average is taken over potentially all combinations of k variables from the full model depending on the model fit for the bootstrap samples $\mathcal{L}_b^*$, not only those showing up in ζ_k. Hence part of the advantage of model selection, namely to obtain a less complex predictor, may be compromised by model averaging.

8.4 PREDICTION ERROR OF THE PITE

The prediction error of the PITE can be defined as

$$\mathrm{PEP}(\mathcal{L}) = E[\{Y(\mathbf{X}_0, 1) - Y(\mathbf{X}_0, 0)$$
$$- (\eta(\mathbf{X}_0, 1, \mathcal{L}) - \eta(\mathbf{X}_0, 0, \mathcal{L}))\}^2]. \quad (8.8)$$

It follows from the Cauchy–Schwartz inequality that

$$\mathrm{PEP}(\mathcal{L}) = E[\{Y(\mathbf{X}_0, 1) - \eta(\mathbf{X}_0, 1, \mathcal{L})\}^2]$$
$$+ E[\{Y(\mathbf{X}_0, 0) - \eta(\mathbf{X}_0, 0, \mathcal{L})\}^2]$$
$$- 2E[\{Y(\mathbf{X}_0, 1) - \eta(\mathbf{X}_0, 1, \mathcal{L})\}$$

$$\times \{Y(\mathbf{X}_0, 0) - \eta(\mathbf{X}_0, 0, \mathcal{L})\}]$$
$$\leq E[\{Y(\mathbf{X}_0, 1) - \eta(\mathbf{X}_0, 1, \mathcal{L})\}^2]$$
$$+ E[\{Y(\mathbf{X}_0, 0) - \eta(\mathbf{X}_0, 0, \mathcal{L})\}^2]$$
$$- 2\sqrt{E[\{Y(\mathbf{X}_0, 1) - \eta(\mathbf{X}_0, 1, \mathcal{L})\}^2]}$$
$$\times \sqrt{E[\{Y(\mathbf{X}_0, 0) - \eta(\mathbf{X}_0, 0, \mathcal{L})\}^2]}.$$
(8.9)

Since a subject is either receiving treatment 0 or treatment 1, $Y(\mathbf{X}, 0)$ and $Y(\mathbf{X}, 1)$ cannot be observed for the same individual. Consequently, the correlation between $Y(0)$ and $Y(1)$ cannot be obtained from the data and mainly an upper bound for the PEP in (8.8) is available. In fact

$$\frac{\sum_{n=1}^{N} t_n (y_n - \eta(\mathbf{x}_n, t_n, \mathcal{L}))^2}{\sum_{n=1}^{N} t_n} \quad \text{and}$$
$$\frac{\sum_{n=1}^{N} (1 - t_n)(y_n - \eta(\mathbf{x}_n, t_n, \mathcal{L}))^2}{\sum_{n=1}^{N} (1 - t_n)} \quad (8.10)$$

are the apparent error estimates of

$$E[\{Y(\mathbf{X}_0, 1) - \eta(\mathbf{X}_0, 1, \mathcal{L})\}^2] \quad \text{and}$$
$$E[\{Y(\mathbf{X}_0, 0) - \eta(\mathbf{X}_0, 0, \mathcal{L})\}^2]$$

respectively. The optimism in these estimators can be reduced by the procedures mentioned previously.

One can do a little more for predictors of a specific class including linear predictors (Tian et al., 2014). Let $\mathbf{W} : \mathcal{R}^K \to \mathcal{R}^K$ be a function of the baseline covariates $\mathbf{X}$, which always includes an intercept. Let $P[T = 1] = p$ for $0 < p < 1$. We consider predictors of the form

$$\eta(\mathbf{x}, t, \mathcal{L}) = \hat{\gamma}(\mathcal{L})'\mathbf{W}(\mathbf{x}) + t\hat{\delta}(\mathcal{L})'\mathbf{W}(\mathbf{x})$$

where $\hat{\gamma}(\mathcal{L})$ and $\hat{\delta}(\mathcal{L})$ minimize

$$\sum_{n=1}^{N} (y_n - \gamma'\mathbf{W}(\mathbf{x}_n) + t_n\delta'\mathbf{W}(\mathbf{x}_n))^2. \quad (8.11)$$

In this simple predictor, the interaction term $t\delta'\mathbf{W}(\mathbf{x})$ reflects the heterogeneous treatment effect across the population. Then the PITE for a future subject $\mathbf{x}_0$ is predicted by

$$\hat{D}(\mathbf{x}_0, \mathcal{L}) = \eta(\mathbf{x}_0, 1, \mathcal{L}) - \eta(\mathbf{x}_0, 0, \mathcal{L}) = \hat{\delta}(\mathcal{L})'\mathbf{W}(\mathbf{x}_0).$$

On the other hand, noting the identity

$$E_P\left[Y\left(\frac{T}{p} - \frac{1-T}{1-p}\right) \bigg| \mathbf{X} = \mathbf{x}\right]$$
$$= \frac{1}{p}E_P[Y|\mathbf{X} = \mathbf{x}, T = 1]P[T = 1]$$
$$- \frac{1}{1-p}E_P[Y|\mathbf{X} = \mathbf{x}, T = 0]P[T = 0]$$
$$= E_P[Y|\mathbf{X} = \mathbf{x}, T = 1] - E_P[Y|\mathbf{X} = \mathbf{x}, T = 0]$$
$$= D(\mathbf{x})$$

one can estimate δ by directly minimizing

$$\sum_{n=1}^{N} \left\{y_n\left(\frac{t_n}{p} - \frac{1-t_n}{1-p}\right) - \delta'\mathbf{W}(\mathbf{x}_n)\right\}^2. \quad (8.12)$$

Prediction Error of the PITE

The multivariate regression (8.11) and the modified outcome estimators (8.12) converge to the same non-random limit δ^*. Furthermore, $\mathbf{W}(\mathbf{x})'\hat{\delta}$ is a sensible estimator for the interaction effect within the class $\mathcal{F} = \{\delta'\mathbf{W}(\mathbf{x}); \delta \in \mathcal{R}^K\}$ by minimizing

$$E_P[(D(\mathbf{X}) = f(\mathbf{X}))^2] \text{ subject to } f \in \mathcal{F}.$$

How is the prediction error of the PITE from (8.8) related to the modified outcome model? Recall that $Y = TY(1) + (1 - T)Y(0)$, which implies

$$Y\left(\frac{T}{p} - \frac{1-T}{1-p}\right) = \frac{TY(1)}{p} - \frac{(1-T)Y(0)}{1-p}.$$

Hence

$$\left(Y\left(\frac{T}{p} - \frac{1-T}{1-p}\right) - D(\mathbf{X})\right)^2$$

$$= \frac{TY(1)^2}{p^2} + \frac{(1-T)Y(0)^2}{(1-p)^2}$$

$$- 2D(\mathbf{X})\left(\frac{TY(1)}{p} - \frac{(1-T)Y(0)}{1-p}\right) + D(\mathbf{X})^2$$

and therefore

$$E\left[\left(Y\left(\frac{T}{p} - \frac{1-T}{1-p}\right) - D(\mathbf{X})\right)^2\right]$$

$$= E[(Y(1) - Y(0) - D(\mathbf{X}))^2]$$

$$+ \frac{1-p}{p}E[Y(1)^2] + \frac{p}{1-p}E[Y(0)^2]$$
$$+ 2E[Y(0)Y(1)].$$

Again, using the Cauchy–Schwartz inequality,

$$\text{PEP}(\mathcal{L}) \leq E\left[\left(Y\left(\frac{T}{p} - \frac{1-T}{1-p}\right) - D(\mathbf{X})\right)^2\right]$$
$$- \frac{1-p}{p}E[Y(1)^2] - \frac{p}{1-p}E[Y(0)^2]$$
$$+ 2\sqrt{E[Y(0)^2]E[Y(1)^2]}. \qquad (8.13)$$

The equations above simplify for $p = 1/2$:

$$\text{PEP}(\mathcal{L})$$
$$= E[(2(2T-1)Y - D(\mathbf{X}))^2] - E[(Y(0) + Y(1))^2]$$
$$\leq E[(2(2T-1)Y - D(\mathbf{X}))^2] - E[Y(0) + Y(1)]^2$$
$$\qquad (8.14)$$

where the second line follows from Jensen's inequality. Hence the apparent error of the PITE estimator $\hat{D}(\mathbf{x})$ for the linear interaction prediction model above is

$$\frac{1}{N}\sum_{n=1}^{N}\left\{y_n\left(\frac{t_n}{p} - \frac{1-t_n}{1-p}\right) - \hat{\delta}'\mathbf{W}(\mathbf{x}_n)\right\}^2$$

plus the estimators of the correction terms in equations (8.13) or (8.14) above.

For predictors of the form

$$\eta(\mathbf{x}, t, \mathcal{L}, \zeta) = \hat{\gamma}(\mathcal{L}, \zeta)'\mathbf{W}(\mathbf{x}) + t\hat{\delta}(\mathcal{L}, \zeta)'\mathbf{W}(\mathbf{x})$$

where $\hat{\gamma}_i(\mathcal{L}, \zeta) = \hat{\delta}_i(\mathcal{L}, \zeta) = 0$ for $i \notin \zeta$, one can estimate an upper bound $\widehat{\text{PEPu}}$ for the prediction error of the PITE in (8.13) or (8.14) for $\zeta_1, \ldots, \zeta_K$ using the regular bootstrap and to choose submodel ζ_k such that

$$\widehat{\text{PEPu}}(\mathcal{L}, \zeta_k) = \min_{k'} \widehat{\text{PEPu}}(\mathcal{L}, \zeta_{k'}).$$

We provide an example of this approach in the Alzheimer case study in the following section.

8.5 A CASE STUDY

The dataset referenced in Schnell et al. (2016) was used in the previous chapter. Here we investigate a linear predictor of severity change based on the values of the four biomarkers: disease severity, age, sex, and a genetic marker contained in the dataset, such that the predictor reads

$$E[Y] = \alpha + \beta t + \sum_{k=1}^{4} \gamma_k x_k + t \sum_{k=1}^{4} \delta_k x_k$$

and would like to get an idea of the precision of this prediction model. Note that in this case

$$D(\mathbf{x}) = \beta + \sum_{k=1}^{4} \delta_k x_k.$$

As discussed in Section 8.2, we estimate the relevant parameters β and δ_k by minimizing the mean residual squared error (RSE)

$$\frac{1}{41}\sum_{n=1}^{41}\{2(2t_n-1)y_n-D(\mathbf{x}_n)\}^2$$

$$=\frac{1}{41}\sum_{n=1}^{41}\left\{2(2t_n-1)y_n-\beta-\sum_{k=1}^{4}\delta_k x_{nk}\right\}^2$$

assuming $p = 1/2$. The parameter estimates are shown in Table 8.1. Since the correction terms in Equation (8.14) are negligible in this example, the upper bound of the apparent error is taken as the obtained minimum of the mean RSE, which equals 62.93. To compensate for the optimism of this estimator we run 1000 bootstrap samples to obtain a correction of 17.32, resulting in a prediction error estimate of 80.25. For comparison, the maximum bound calculated from (8.9) is 104.11.

Table 8.1 Parameter estimates of linear predictor for Alzheimer data

Parameter	Marker	Estimate	StdErr
β		−14.518442	12.42435
δ_1	Severity	−0.016837	0.161010
δ_2	Age	0.286140	0.153540
δ_3	Carrier(Y)	−1.015439	2.672602
δ_4	Sex(M)	−5.513353	2.754234

This looks unacceptably high considering that the severity is in the range 10–45.

Considering the standardized estimates, age and sex seem to be the most influential markers. Male patients are predicted to have an extra gain of 5 units on the severity scale under test treatment as compared to female patients, while one year of age cuts the efficacy of the test treatment by about 0.3 units. Indeed if one conducts a forward variable selection that enters variables as long as the BIC decreases, age and sex are retained in the model.

Table 8.2 shows the prediction errors of the PITE for models with one to four variables as determined by forward selection. The optimism is calculated from 1000 bootstrap samples. It turns out that for the Alzheimer data the PITE is most accurate for predictors with two variables. Noteworthy is the trade-off between RSE, which decreases, and optimism, which increases with the number of variables in the model.

Table 8.2 Upper bounds of the prediction error estimate of the PITE for predictors with one to four variables for the Alzheimer data

No. of variables	Mean RSE	Optimism	$\widehat{PEPu}$
1	69.39	13.15	82.54
2	63.20	15.02	78.22
3	62.95	16.72	79.67
4	62.93	17.32	80.25

Table 8.3 Selection percentage of variables for the Alzheimer data for a predictor with two variables

Variables in model	Selection (%)
Age, sex	59.9
Sex, severity	10.7
Age, severity	9.8
Age, carrier	8.3
Sex, carrier	8.2
Carrier, severity	3.1
Sex	78.8
Age	78.0

Table 8.3 displays how often two specific variables arose in the predictors from the 1000 bootstrap samples. As mentioned earlier, the averaged predictor contains not only age and sex as obtained from forward selection but potentially all variables from the full model. In fact, age or sex are selected in about 78% of the samples, but in combination only in about 60%. Severity is selected with age or sex in more than 20% and carrier in more than 16% of the samples.

8.6 CONCLUDING REMARKS

We have seen that data modeling plays an important role in subgroup analysis. Modeling offers the use of the size of interactions between treatment and covariates to give information about subgroups in a dataset instead of relying on within-group comparisons. On the flip side there is the risk that the size of interactions is not only data driven but is also affected by modeling. Since all models are known to be wrong (Box, 1976), this raises the question to what extent the results of the modeling exercise are reliable. Goodness-of-fit and residual analysis may not be able to address the issue satisfactorily. Work by Bickel et al. (2006) shows that goodness-of-fit tests have very little power unless the direction of the alternative is precisely specified. This implies that omnibus goodness-of-fit tests will have little power and will not reject until the lack of fit is extreme.

Following Breiman (2001), the most obvious way to see how well a model emulates nature is this: treat a new case $\mathbf{X}_0 = \mathbf{x}_0$ with treatment $T = t_0$ to observe an outcome Y_0. Then put the same case down the model and obtain $\eta(\mathbf{x}_0, t_0)$. The closeness of Y_0 and $\eta(\mathbf{x}_0, t_0)$ is a measure how well the model fits. For a data model this translates as: fit the parameters in your model by using your data, then, using the data, fit the model, predict the data, and see how good your prediction is. If the model has too many parameters it may give an overoptimistic estimate of accuracy. However, as we saw, there are methods to remove this bias.

Although the prediction error of the outcome for a specific treatment given the covariates can be obtained, estimating the prediction error of the potential effect difference under alternative treatments – the PITE – faces some intrinsic problems. Because each subject can only be administered one of the alternative treatments, the correlation between the potential outcomes is not estimable but only upper bounds can be provided. In this chapter we made a first attempt in this direction.

9

Outlook

Just because a technique is widely used it does not mean that it is valuable. And just because there is little theoretical evidence validating a method does not mean it is not valid.

William F. Rosenberger and Olexandr Sverdlov
(Rosenberger and Sverdlov, 2008)

This chapter brings our subgroup analysis journey to a stop, surely not to an end. The topic is a rapidly expanding field of research, as is indicated by the number of new articles being published. As said at the beginning, a presentation of a broad topic like subgroup analyses is influenced by the preferences and experience of the presenter and will hardly be exhaustive. Nevertheless it is hoped that the reader of this book got an understanding of the different aspects of the matter. The final chapter shall briefly go over topics or approaches that have not been mentioned or treated so far.

From a methodology perspective, subgroup analysis draws on different areas of statistics, a major one being statistical modeling. In this book we built on the classical regression models like (generalized) linear models and the proportional hazards model for survival data. Some readers may regret that non-parametric regression or regression using fractional polynomials as described in Royston and Sauerbrei (2008) are not mentioned. A similar concern may be raised in regard to Bayesian methods. In defense of the author it can be said that there is a full chapter on hierarchical modeling within an empirical Bayesian framework that can be translated into a fully Bayesian presentation. Also, neural nets and other machine learning methods are not mentioned.

This does not mean that these methods offer no value over the procedures described, though new is not always better. For example, systematic reviews do not support better performance of machine learning methods over logistic regression for clinical prediction models (Christodoulou et al., 2019). In the end, what is important is that the objectives of subgroup analysis are addressed appropriately. Methods are to some extent interchangeable and no method works best under any circumstances.

To obtain subgroups from continuous covariates, their range has to be split by a cutpoint that can either be pre-defined or optimized from the data. The latter may result in better prediction; however, there is the disadvantage that the next dataset may result in a different cutpoint, which makes comparisons difficult. Nevertheless these methods, also known as recursive partitioning algorithms, have been successfully applied in practice (Hothorn et al., 2006; X Su et al., 2009; Lipkovich et al., 2011; Lipkovich and Dmitrienko, 2014).

The book emphasizes applications with relatively few biomarkers or covariates, mainly in the order of 10 to 30. Some of the methods presented also apply to high dimensional problems where the number of covariates exceeds the number of subjects. This is not only true for the LASSO, but also for forward selection, as demonstrated in an example for hierarchical models.

When subgroup analyses are done after selection, selection has to be accounted for in the analysis, otherwise estimates will be unstable and biased and confidence intervals will not attain the required coverage. What is meant by coverage in the context of selection can depend on different concepts like post-selection inference (Berk et al., 2013) or selective inference (Taylor and Tibshirani, 2015; Lee et al., 2016; Taylor and Tibshirani, 2017), as discussed in Leeb et al. (2015), Bachoc et al. (2019).

Regarding software, most of the case studies presented in this book have been analyzed using SAS Version 9.4 (SAS, 2016) with the exception of some of the examples in Chapter 7 using R. The bootstrap method to account for selection bias is implemented in an R package called subtee (Ballarini et al., 2019) together with a model averaging algorithm from Bornkamp et al. (2017).

Bibliography

H Akaike. Formation theory and an extension of the maximum likelihood principle. In B N Petrov and F Csaki, editors, *Second International Symposium on Information Theory*, pages 267–281. Budapest, HU: Akademiai Kiado, 1973.

M Alosh, K Fritsch, M Huque, K Mahjoob, G Pennello, M Rothmann, E Russek-Cohen, F Smith, and S Wilson. Statistical considerations on subgroup analysis in clinical trials. *Statistics in Biopharmaceutical Research*, 7:286–304, 2015.

M Alosh, M F Huque, F Bretz, and R B D'Agostino. Tutorial on statistical considerations on subgroup analyses in confirmatory clinical trials. *Statistics in Medicine*, 36:1334–1360, 2017.

Antiplatelet Trialists' Collaboration. Collaborative overview of randomised trials of antiplatelet therapy. I: Prevention of death, myocardial infarction, and stroke by prolonged antiplatelet therapy in various categories of patients. *British Medical Journal*, 308:81–106, 1994.

S F Assmann, S J Pocock, L E Enos, and L E Kasten. Subgroup analyses and other (mis)uses of baseline data in clinical trials. *Lancet*, 355:1064–1069, 2000.

P C Austin and L J Brunner. Inflation of the type I error rate when a continuous confounding variable is categorized in logistic regression analysis. *Statistics in Medicine*, 23:1159–1178, 2004.

F Bachoc, H Leeb, and B M Pötscher. Valid confidence intervals for post-model-selection predictors. *The Annals of Statistics*, 47:1475–1504, 2019.

N M Ballarini, G K Rosenkranz, T Jaki, F König, and M Posch. Subgroup identification in clinical trials via the predicted individual effect. *PLoS ONE*, 13:e0205971, 2018.

N M Ballarini, M Thomas, G K Rosenkranz, and B Bornkamp. subtee: An R package for subgroup analyses in clinical trials. *Journal of Statistical Software (submitted)*, 0:0–0, 2019.

T A Ban. The role of serendipity in drug discovery. *Dialogues in Clinical Neuroscience*, 8:335–344, 2006.

B Bannwarth and F Berenbaum. Lumiracoxib in the management of osteoarthritis and acute pain. *Expert Opinion on Pharmacotherapy*, 8: 1551–1564, 2007.

E O Bayman, K Chaloner, and M K Cowles. Detecting qualitative interaction: A Bayesian approach. *Statistics in Medicine*, 29:455–463, 2010.

R Bender, A Koch, G Skipka, T Kaiser, and S Lange. No inconsistent trial assessments by NICE and IQWiG: different assessment goals may lead to different assessment results regarding subgroup analyses. *Journal of Clinical Epidemiology*, 63:1305–1307, 2010.

J O Berger, X Wang, and L Shen. A Bayesian approach to subgroup identification. *Journal of Biopharmaceutical Statistics*, 24:110–129, 2014.

R Berk, L Brown, A Buja, K Zhang, and L Zhao. Valid post-selection inference. *Annals of Statistics*, 41:802–837, 2013.

P Bickel, Y Ritov, and T Stoker. Taylor-made tests for goodness-of-fit for semiparametric hypotheses. *Annals of Statistics*, 34:721–741, 2006.

JG Booth and JP Hobert. Standard errors of prediction in generalized linear mixed models. *Journal of the American Statistical Association*, 93:262–272, 1998.

B Bornkamp, D Ohlssen, B P Magnusson, and H Schmidli. Model averaging for treatment effect estimation in subgroups. *Pharmaceutical Statistics*, 16: 133–142, 2017.

G E P Box. Science and statistics. *Journal of the American Statistical Association*, 71:791–799, 1976.

A Bradford Hill. Reflections on the controlled trial. *Annals of Rheumatoid Diseases*, 25:107–113, 1966.

L Breiman. *Probability*. Addison-Wesley Pub. Co., Reading, Mass., 1968.

L Breiman. Bagging predictors. *Machine Learning*, 24:123–140, 1996.

L Breiman. Statistical modeling: The two cultures. *Statistical Science*, 16: 199–231, 2001.

L Breiman and P Spector. Submodel selection and evaluation in regression. The X-random case. *International Statistical Review*, 60:291–319, 1992.

ST Brookes, E Whitely, TJ Peters, PA Mulheran, M Egger, and GD Smith. Subgroup analyses in randomized trials: quantifying the risks of false positives and false negatives. *Health Technology Assessments*, 33:1–51, 2001.

ST Brookes, E Whitely, M Egger, GD Smith, PA Mulheran, and TJ Peters. Subgroup analyses in randomized trials: risks of subgroup analyses; power and sample size for the interaction test. *Journal of Clinical Epidemiology*, 57: 229–236, 2004.

D Buck and B Hemmer. Biomarkers of treatment response in multiple sclerosis. *Expert Review of Neurotherapeutics*, 14:165–172, 2014.

P Bühlmann and B Yu. Analyzing bagging. *Annals of Statistics*, 30:927–961, 2002.

M Buyse and I C Marschner. Assessment of statistical heterogeneity in the PLATO trial. *Cardiology*, 118:138, 2011.

D Byar and S Green. The choice of treatment for cancer patients based on covariate information: application to prostate cancer. *Bulletin du Cancer*, 67: 477–490, 1980.

T Cai, L Tian, P H Wong, and L J Wei. Analysis of randomized comparative clinical trial data for personalized treatment selections. *Biostatistics*, 12: 270–282, 2011.

CAPRIE Steering Committee. A randomised, blinded, trial of clopidogrel versus aspirin in patients at risk of ischaemic events (CAPRIE). *Lancet*, 348: 1329–1339, 1996.

B P Carlin and T A Louis. Empirical Bayes: Past, present and future. *Journal of the American Statistical Association*, 95:1286–1289, 2000.

B P Carlin and T A Louis. *Bayesian Methods for Data Analysis*. Chapman and Hall/CRC, 2009.

C H Chen and S L George. The bootstrap and identification of prognostic factors via Cox's proportional hazards regression model. *Statistics in Medicine*, 4: 39–46, 1985.

S Chen, L Tian, T Cai, and M Yu. A general statistical framework for subgroup identification and comparative treatment scoring. *Biometrics*, 73:1199–1209, 2017.

E Christodoulou, J Ma, G S Collins, E W Steyerberg, J Y Verbakel, and B van Calster. A systematic review shows no performance benefit of machine learning over logistic regression for clinical prediction models. *Journal of Clinical Epidemiology*, 110:12–22, 2019.

A Cohen and H Sackrowitz. Two-stage conditionally unbiased estimators of the selected normal means. *Statistics and Probability Letters*, 8:273–278, 1989.

G A Colditz, T F Brewer, C S Berkey, M E Wilson, E Burdick, H V Fineberg, and F Mosteller. Efficacy of BCG vaccine in the prevention of tuberculosis. *Journal of the American Medical Association*, 271:698–702, 1994.

D R Cox. Regression models and life tables. *Journal of the Royal Statistical Society B*, 34:187–220, 1972.

D R Cox. Partial likelihood. *Biometrika*, 62:269–276, 1975.

F Cumsille, S I Bangdiwala, P K Sen, and L L Kupper. Effect of dichotomizing a continuous variable on the model structure in multiple linear regression models. *Communications in Statistics—Theory and Methods*, 29:643–654, 2000.

S Dalal and W Hall. Approximating priors by mixtures of natural conjugate priors. *Journal of the Royal Statistical Society, Series B*, 45:278–286, 1983.

A Dane, A Spencer, G Rosenkranz, I Lipkovich, and T Parke. Subgroup analysis and interpretation for phase 3 confirmatory trials: White paper of the EFSPI/PSI working group on subgroup analysis. *Pharmaceutical Statistics*, 18:126–139, 2019.

C E Davis and D P Leffingwell. Empirical Bayes estimates of subgroup effects in clinical trials. *Controlled Clinical Trials*, 11:37–42, 1990.

A P Dempster, N M Laird, and D B Rubin. Maximum likelihood from incomplete data via the EM algorithm (with discussion). *Journal of the Royal Statistical Society B*, 39:1–38, 1977.

R DerSimonian and N Laird. Meta-analysis in clinical trials. *Controlled Clinical Trials*, 7:177–188, 1986.

P J Diggle, P J Heagerty, K-Y Liang, and S L Zeger. *Analysis of Longitudinal Data*. Oxford University Press, 2nd edition, 2002.

W DuMouchel. Bayesian data mining in large frequency tables, with an application to the FDA spontaneous reporting system. *The American Statistician*, 53:177–190, 1999.

B Efron. Bootstrap methods: another look at the jackknife. *Annals of Statistics*, 7:1–26, 1979.

B Efron. Censored data and the bootstrap. *Journal of the American Statistical Association*, 76:312–319, 1981.

B Efron. Estimating the error rate of a prediction rule: some improvements on cross-validation. *Journal of the American Statistical Association*, 78:316–331, 1983.

B Efron. Size, power and false discovery rates. *Annals of Statistics*, 35: 1351–1377, 2007.

B Efron. Tweedie's formula and selection bias. *Journal of the American Statistical Association*, 106:1602–1614, 2011.

B Efron. Estimation and accuracy after model selection. *Journal of the American Statistical Association*, 109:991–1007, 2014.

B Efron and C Morris. Stein's estimation rule and its competitors - an empirical Bayes approach. *Journal of the American Statistical Association*, 68:117–130, 1973.

B Efron and C Morris. Data analysis using Stein's estimator and its generalizations. *Journal of the American Statistical Association*, 70:311–319, 1975.

B Efron and R Tibshirani. Bootstrap methods for standard errors, confidence intervals, and other measures of statistical accuracy. *Statistical Science*, 1: 54–77, 1986.

B Efron and R Tibshirani. *An Introduction to the Bootstrap*. Chapman and Hall/CRC, 1993.

B Efron and R Tibshirani. Improvements on cross-validation: the .632+ bootstrap method. *Journal of the American Statistical Association*, 92: 548–560, 1997.

EMA. *Guideline on the investigation of subgroups in confirmatory clinical trials*. European Medicines Agency, 2019.

J Fan, F Song, and M O Bachmann. Justification and reporting of subgroup analyses were lacking or inadequate in randomized controlled trials. *Journal of Clinical Epidemiology*, 108:17–25, 2019.

M E Farkouh, H Kirshner, R A Harrington, S Ruland, F W A Verheugt, T J Schnitzer, G T Burmester, E Mysler, M C Hochberg, M Doherty, E Ehrsam, X Gitton, G Krammer, B Mellein, A Gimona, P Matchaba, C J Hawkey, and J H Chesebro on behalf of the TARGET Study Group. Comparison of lumiracoxib with naproxen and ibuprofen in the Therapeutic Arthritis Research and Gastrointestinal Event Trial (TARGET), cardiovascular outcomes: randomised controlled trial. *Lancet*, 364:675–684, 2004.

M R Farlow, G W Small, P Quarg, and A Krause. Efficacy of rivastigmine in Alzheimer's disease patients with rapid disease progression: Results of a meta-analysis. *Dementia and Geriatric Cognitive Disorders*, 20:192–197, 2005.

FDA. *Content and Format of a New Drug Application*. Food and Drug Administration, 1988.

FDA. *Drug Approval Package: Plavix/Clopidogrel bisulfate*. Food and Drug Administration, 1997.

FDA. *Paving the Way for Personalized Medicine*. Food and Drug Administration, 2013.

FDA. *FDA Action Plan to Enhance the Collection and Availability of Demographic Subgroup Data*. Food and Drug Administration, 2014.

FDA. *Personalized Medicine at FDA—2017 Progress Report*. Food and Drug Administration, 2017.

AR Feinstein. The problem of cogent subgroups: A clinicostatistical tragedy. *Journal of Clinical Epidemiology*, 51:297–299, 1998.

J Friedman, T Hastie, and R Tibshirani. Regularization paths for generalized linear models via coordinate descent. *Journal of Statistical Software*, 33:1–22, 2010.

N B Gabler, N Duan, E Raneses, L Suttner, M Ciarametaro, E Cooney, R W Dubois, S D Halpern, and R L Kravitz. No improvement in the reporting of clinical trial subgroup effects in high-impact general medical journals. *Trials*, 17:1–12, 2016.

M A Gaglia and R Waksman. Overview of the 2010 Food and Drug Administration Cardiovascular and Renal Drugs Advisory Committee Meeting regarding ticagrelor. *Circulation*, 123:451–456, 2011.

M Gail and R Simon. Testing for qualitative interactions between treatment effects and patient subsets. *Biometrics*, 41:361–372, 1985.

M H Gail, S Wieand, and S Piantadosi. Biased estimates of treatment effect in randomized experiments with non-linear regressions and omitted covariates. *Biometrika*, 71:431–444, 1984.

GISSI Study Group. Effectiveness of intravenous thrombolytic treatment in acute myocardial infarction. *Lancet*, 1:397–401, 1986.

S Greenland. Principles of multilevel modelling. *International Journal of Epidemiology*, 29:158–167, 2000.

J-M Grouin, M Coste, and J Lewis. Subgroup analyses in randomized clinical trials: statistical and regulatory issues. *Journal of Biopharmaceutical Statistics*, 15:869–882, 2005.

F Guillemin. Primer: the fallacy of subgroup analyses. *Nature Clinical Practice Rheumatology*, 3:407–413, 2007.

E Hargrave-Thomas, B Yu, and J Reynisson. Serendipity in anticancer drug discovery. *World Journal of Clinical Oncology*, 3:1–6, 2012.

J Hasford, P Bramlage, G Koch, W Lehmacher, K Einhäupl, and PM Rothwell. Inconsistent trial assessments by the National Institute for Health and Clinical Excellence and IQWiG: standards for the performance and interpretation of subgroup analyses are needed. *Journal of Clinical Epidemiology*, 63: 1298–1304, 2010.

J Hasford, P Bramlage, G Koch, W Lehmacher, K Einhäupl, and PM Rothwell. Letter to the editor: Standards for subgroup analysis are needed?—we couldn't agree more. *Journal of Clinical Epidemiology*, 64:451, 2011.

T Hastie, R Tibshirani, and Wainwright M. *Statistical Learning with Sparsity*. CRC Press, Boca Raton, 2015.

W W Hauck, S Anderson, and S M Marcus. Should we adjust for covariates in non-linear regression analyses of randomized clinical trials? *Controlled Clinical Trials*, 19:249–256, 1998.

G Heinze, C Wallisch, and D Dunkler. Variable selection – a review and recommendations for the practicing statistician. *Biometrical Journal*, 60: 431–449, 2018.

J Z Hines, P Lurie, and S M Wolfe. Post hoc analysis does not establish effectiveness of rTMS for depression. *Neuropsychopharmacology*, 34: 2053–2054, 2009.

R Horton. From star signs to trial guidelines. *Lancet*, 355:1033–1034, 2000.

R I Horwitz, B H Singer, R W Markuch, and C M Viscoli. Can treatment that is helpful on average be harmful to some patients? A study of conflicting information needs of clinical inquiry and drug regulation. *Journal of Clinical Epidemiology*, 49:395–400, 1996.

R I Horwitz, B H Singer, R W Markuch, and C M Viscoli. On reaching the tunnel at the end of the light. *Journal of Clinical Epidemiology*, 50:753–755, 1997.

T Hothorn, K Hornik, and A Zeileis. Unbiased recursive partitioning: A conditional inference framework. *Journal of Computational and Graphical Statistics*, 15:651–674, 2006.

G W Imbens and D B Rubin. *Causal Inference for Statistics, Social, and Biomedical Sciences*. Cambridge University Press, 2015.

ISIS–2 Collaborative Group. Randomised trial of intravenous streptokinase, oral aspirin, both or neither among 17187 cases of suspected acute myocardial infarction: ISIS–2. *Lancet*, pages 349–360, 1988.

W James and C Stein. Estimation with quadratic loss. *Proceedings of the Fourth Berkeley Symposium on Mathematical Statistics and Probability*, pages 361–379, 1961.

H E Jones, D I Ohlssen, B Neuenschwander, A Racine, and M Branson. Bayesian models for subgroup analysis in clinical trials. *Clinical Trials*, 8:129–143, 2011.

D J Jonker, C J O'Callaghan, C S Karapetis, J R Zalcberg, D Tu, H J Au, S R Berry, M Krahn, T Price, R J Simes, N C Tebbutt, G van Hazel, R Wierzbicki, C Langer, and M J Moore. Cetuximab for the treatment of colorectal cancer. *New England Journal of Medicine*, 357:2040–2048, 2007.

D Kahneman. *Thinking, fast and slow*. Penguin Books Ltd., London, 2012.

C Karapetis, S Khambata-Ford, D Jonker, C O'CCallaghan, D Tu, N Tebbut, J Simes, H Chalchal, J Shapiro, S Robitaille, S Price, L Sheperd, H Au, C Langer, M Moore, and J Zalcberg. K-ras mutations and benefit from cetuximab in advanced colorectal cancer. *New England Journal of Medicine*, 359:1757–1765, 2008.

RE Kass and D Steffey. Approximate Bayesian inference in conditionally independent hierarchical models (parametric empirical Bayes models). *Journal of the American Statistical Association*, 84:717–726, 1989.

D Kivaranovic and H Leeb. Expected length of post-model-selection predictors. *arXiv preprint*, arXiv:1803.01665, 2018.

A Krause and J Pinheiro. Modeling and simulation to adjust *p*-values in presence of regression to the mean effect. *The American Statistician*, 61: 302–307, 2007.

S W Lagakos. The challenge of subgroup analyses—reporting without distorting. *New England Journal of Medicine*, 354:1667–1669, 2006.

A Lamont, MD Lyons, T Jaki, E Stuart, DJ Feaster, K Tharmaratnam, D Oberski, H Ishwaran, DK Wilson, and ML Van Hoorn. Identification of predicted individual treatment effects in randomized clinical trials. *Statistical Methods in Medical Research*, 27:142–157, 2018.

J D Lee, D L Sun, Y Sun, and J E Taylor. Exact post-selection inference, with application to the lasso. *The Annals of Statistics*, 44:907–927, 2016.

J J Lee and D B Rubin. Evaluating the validity of post-hoc subgroup inferences: a case study. *The American Statistician*, 70:39–46, 2016.

H Leeb, B M Pötscher, and K Ewald. On various confidence intervals post-model-selection. *Statistical Science*, 30:216–227, 2015.

KR Lees, JA Zivin, T Ashwood, A Davalos, SM Davis, HC Diener, J Grotta, P Lyden, A Shuaib, HG Hårdemark, WW Wasiewski, and Stroke-Acute Ischemic NXY Treatment (SAINT I) Trial Investigators. NXY-059 for acute ischemic stroke. *New England Journal of Medicine*, 354:588–600, 2006.

Z Li, C Chuang-Stein, and C Hoseyni. The probability of observing negative subgroup results when the treatment effect is positive and homogeneous across all subgroups. *Drug Information Journal*, 41:47–56, 2007.

I Lipkovich and A Dmitrienko. Strategies for identifying predictive biomarkers and subgroups with enhanced treatment effect in clinical trials using SIDES. *Journal of Biopharmaceutical Statistics*, 24:130–153, 2014.

I Lipkovich, A Dmitrienko, J Denne, and G Enas. Subgroup identification based on differential effect search—a recursive partitioning method for establishing response to treatment in patient subpopulations. *Statistics in Medicine*, 30: 2601–2621, 2011.

S H Lisanby, M M Husain, P B Rosenquist, D Maixner, R Gutierrez, A Krystal, William Gilmer, L B Marangell, S Aaronson, Z J Daskalakis, R Canterbury, E Richelson, H A Sackeim, and M S George. Daily left prefrontal repetitive transcranial magnetic stimulation in the acute treatment of major depression: clinical predictors of outcome in a multisite, randomized controlled clinical trial. *Neuropsychopharmacology*, 34:522–534, 2009.

M Lonergan, S J Senn, C McNamee, A K Daly, R Sutton, A Hattersley, E Pearson, and M Pirmohamed. Defining drug response for stratified medicine. *Drug Discovery Today*, 22:173–179, 2017.

P McCullagh and J P Nelder. *Generalized Linear Models*. Chapman and Hall, 2nd edition, 1989.

P A McCullough, M E Bertraud, J A Brinker, and F Stacul. A meta-analysis of the renal safety of isosmolar iodixanol compared with low-osmolar contrast media. *Journal of the American College of Cardiology*, 48:692–699, 2006.

MHLW. *Basic Concepts for Joint International Clinical Trials*. Ministry of Health, Labour and Welfare of Japan, 2007.

G Molenberghs and G Verbeke. *Models for Discrete Longitudinal Data*. Springer Verlag, 2005.

C N Morris. Parametric empirical Bayes inference: theory and application. *Journal of the American Statistical Association*, 78:47–55, 1983.

J D Naranjo and J W McKean. Adjusting for regression effects in uncontrolled studies. *Biometrics*, 57:178–181, 2001.

M R Nester. An applied statistician's creed. *Applied Statistics*, 45:401–410, 1996.

B Neuenschwander, S Wandel, S Roychoudhury, and S Bailey. Robust exchangeability designs for early phase clinical trials with multiple strata. *Pharmaceutical Statistics*, 15: 123–134, 2015.

T Ondra, A Dmitrienko, T Friede, A Graf, F Miller, N Stallard, and M Posch. Methods for identification and confirmation of targeted subgroups: a systematic review. *Journal of Biopharmaceutical Statistics*, 26:99–119, 2016.

J P O'Reardon, H B Solvason, P G Janicak, S Sampson, K E Isenberg, Z Nahas, W M Mcdonald, D Avery, P B Fitzgerals, C Loo, M A Demitrak, M S George, and H A Sackeim. Efficacy and safety of transcranial magnetic stimulation in the acute treatment of major depression: a multisite randomized controlled trial. *Biological Psychiatry*, 62:1208–1216, 2007.

R Peto. Misleading subgroup analyses in GISSI. *The American Journal of Cardiology*, 66:771, 1990.

H Quan, M Li, J Chen, P Gallo, B Binkowitz, E Ibia, Y Tanaka, P Ouyang, X Lue, G Li, S Menjoge, S Talerico, and K Ikeda. Assessment of consistency of treatment effects in multiregional clinical trials. *Drug Information Journal*, 44:619–634, 2010.

G Raghu, K K Brown, W Z Bradford, K Starko, P W Noble, D A Schwartz, and T E King. A placebo–controlled trial of interferon gamma–1b in patients with idiopathic pulmonary fibrosis. *New England Journal of Medicine*, 350: 125–133, 2004.

JS Remington, B Efron, E Cavanaugh, HJ Simon, and A Trejos. Studies on toxoplasmosis as measured by the Sabin-Feldman dye test. *Transactions of the Royal Society of Tropical Medicine and Hygiene*, pages 252–267, 1970.

H Robbins. An empirical Bayes approach to statistics. *Proceedings of the Third Berkeley Symposium on Mathematical Statistics and Probability*, pages 157–163, 1956.

L D Robinson and N P Jewell. Some surprising results about covariate adjustment in logistic regression. *International Statistical Review*, 58:227–240, 1991.

W F Rosenberger and O Sverdlov. Handling covariates in the design of clinical trials. *Statistical Science*, 23:404–419, 2008.

G K Rosenkranz. An approach to integrated safety analyses of clinical trials. *Drug Information Journal*, 44:649–657, 2010.

G K Rosenkranz. Bootstrap corrections of treatment effect estimates following selection. *Computational Statistics & Data Analysis*, 69:220–227, 2014.

G K Rosenkranz. Exploratory subgroup analysis in clinical trials by model selection. *Biometrical Journal*, 58:1217–1228, 2016.

G K Rosenkranz. Can we identify patients at high risk of harm under a generally safe intervention? *International Journal of Clinical Biostatistics and Biometrics*, 3:1–7, 2017.

G K Rosenkranz. Empirical Bayes estimators in hierarchical models with mixture priors. *Journal of Applied Statistics*, 45:2958–2980, 2018.

P M Rothwell. Subgroup analysis in randomised controlled trials: importance, indications, and interpretation. *Lancet*, 365:176–186, 2005.

P Royston and W Sauerbrei. *Multivariable model-building: a pragmatic approach to regression anaylsis based on fractional polynomials for modelling continuous variables.* John Wiley & Sons Ltd.,2008.

P Royston, D G Altman, and W Sauerbrei. Dichotomizing continuous predictors in multiple regression: a bad idea. *Statistics in Medicine*, 25:127–141, 2006.

SAS. *Statistical Analysis System*. SAS Institute Inc., Cary, NC, USA, 2016.

W Sauerbrei. The use of resampling methods to simplify regression models in medical statistics. *Applied Statistics*, 48:313–329, 1999.

W Sauerbrei and M Schumacher. A bootstrap resampling procedure for model building: application to the Cox regression model. *Statistics in Medicine*, 11:2093–2109, 1992.

H Scheffé. A method for judging all contrasts in the analysis of variance. *Biometrika*, 40:87–104, 1953.

H Schmidli, S Gsteiger, S Roychoudhury, A O'Hagan, D Spiegelhalter, and B Neuenschwander. Robust meta-analytic-predictive priors in clinical trials with historical information. *Biometrics*, 70:1023–1032, 2014.

C Schmoor and M Schumacher. Effects of covariate omission and categorization when analyzing randomized trials with the Cox model. *Statistics in Medicine*, 16:225–237, 1997.

P M Schnell, Q Tang, W W Offen, and B P Carlin. A Bayesian credible subgroup approach to identifying patient subgroups with positive treatment effect. *Biometrics*, 72:1026–1036, 2016.

DA Schoenfeld. Sample-size formula for the proportional hazards regression model. *Biometrics*, 39:499–503, 1983.

KF Schulz, DG Altman, for the CONSORT Group D Moher. Consort 2010 statement: updated guidelines for reporting parallel group ranomised trials. *BMJ*, 340:332, 2010.

G Schwartz. Estimating the dimensions of a model. *Annals of Statistics*, 6: 461–464, 1979.

S Senn. Individual therapy: new dawn or false dawn. *Drug Information Journal*, 35:1479–1494, 2001.

S Senn. *Statistical Issues in Drug Development*. John Wiley & Sons Ltd., 2nd edition, 2007.

S Senn. Francis Galton and regression to the mean. *Significance*, 8:124–126, 2011.

S Senn and F Harrell. On wisdom after the event. *Journal of Clinical Epidemiology*, 50:749–751, 1997.

M C Simmonds and J P T Higgins. A general framework for the use of logistic regression models in meta-analysis. *Statistical Methods in Medical Research*, 25:2858–2877, 2016.

J B Singer, S Lewitzky, E Leroy, F Yang, X Zhao, L Klickstein, T M Wright, J Meyer, and A Paulding. A genome-wide study identifies HLA alleles associated with lumiracoxib-related liver injury. *Nature Genetics*, 42:711–716, 2010.

D Singh, PG Febbo, K Ross, DG Jackson, J Manola, C Ladd, P Tamayo, AA Renshaw, AV D'Amico, JP Richie, ES Lander, M Loda, PW Kantoff, TR Golub, and WR Sellers. Gene expresion correlates of clinical prostate cancer behavior. *Cancer Cell*, 1:203–209, 2002.

R E Slager, A O Babatunde, C A Hawkins, Y P Yen, S E Peters, SE Wenzel, D A Meyers, and E R Bleeke. IL-4 receptor polymorphisms predict reduction in asthma exacerbations during response to an anti-IL-4 receptor α antagonist. *Journal of Allergy and Clinical Immunology*, 130:516–522, 2012.

D J Slamon, B Leyland-Jones B, S Shak, H Fuchs, V Paton, A Bajamonde, T Fleming, W Eiermann, J Wolter, M Pegram, J Baselga, and L Norton. Use of chemotherapy plus a monoclonal antibody against HER2 for metastatic breast cancer that overexpresses HER2. *New England Journal of Medicine*, 344: 783–792, 2001.

P Sleight. Debate: Subgroup analysis in clinical trials—fun to look at, but don't believe them. *Current Controlled Trials in Cardiovascular Medicine*, 1:25–27, 2000.

J A Sparano and S Paik. Development of the 21-gene assay and its application in clinical practice and clinical trials. *Journal of Clinical Oncology*, 26:721–728, 2008.

J A Sparano, R J Gray, D F Makower, K I Pritchard, K S Albain, D F Hayes, C E Geyer, E C Dees, E A Perez, J A Olson, J A Zujewski, T Lively, S S Badve, T J Saphner, L I Wagner, T J Whelan, M J Ellis, S Paik, W C Wood, P Ravdin, M M Keane, H L Gomez Moreno, P S Reddy, T F Goggins, I A Meyer, A M Brufsky, D L Toppmeyer, V G Kaklamani, J N Atkins, J L Berenberg, J Abrams, and G W Sledge. Prospective validation of a 21-gene expression assay in breast cancer. *New England Journal of Medicine*, 373:2005–2014, 2015.

J A Sparano, R J Gray, D F Makower, K I Pritchard, K S Albain, D F Hayes, C E Geyer, E C Dees, M P Goetz, J A Olson, T Lively, S S Badve, T J Saphner, L I Wagner, T J Whelan, M J Ellis, S Paik, W C Wood, P M Ravdin, M M Keane, H L Gomez Moreno, P S Reddy, T F Goggins, I A Meyer, A M Brufsky, D L Toppmeyer, V G Kaklamani, J L Berenberg, J Abrams, and G W Sledge. Adjuvant chemotherapy guided by a 21-gene expression assay in breast cancer. *New England Journal of Medicine*, 379:111–121, 2018.

N Stallard, S Todd, and J Whitehead. Estimation following selection of the largest of two normal means. *Journal of Statistical Planning and Inference*, 138: 1629–1638, 2008.

CM Stein. Inadmissibility of the usual estimator for the mean of a multivariate normal distribution. *Proceedings of the Third Berkeley Symposium on Mathematical Statistics and Probability*, pages 197–206, 1956.

E W Steyerberg, F E Harrell, G J J M Borsboom, M J C Eijkemans, Y Vergouwe, and J D F Habbema. Internal validation of predictive models: Efficiency of some procedures for logistic regression analysis. *Journal of Clinical Epidemiology*, 54:774–781, 2001.

M Stone. Cross-validatory choice and assessment of statistica predictions. *Journal of the Royal Statistical Society B*, 36:111–147, 1974.

R Sykes. The pharmaceutical industry in the new millenium: Capturing the scientific promise. pages 1–28. Centre for Medicines Research, 1977.

J Taylor and R Tibshirani. Post-selection inference for ℓ_1 penalized likelihood models. *The Canadian Journal of Statistics*, pages 1–21, 2017.

J Taylor and RJ Tibshirani. Statistical learning and selective inference. *Proceedings of the National Academy of Sciences*, 112:7629–7634, 2015.

The Canadian Cooperative Study Group. A randomised trial of aspirin and sulfinpyrazone in threatened stroke. *New England Journal of Medicine*, 299: 301–314, 1978.

L Tian, AA Alizadeh, AJ Gentles, and R Tibshirani. A simple method for estimating interactions between a treatment and a large number of covariates. *Journal of the American Statistical Association*, 109:1517–1532, 2014.

X Tian and J E Taylor. Selective inference with a randomized response. *Annals of Statistics*, 46:679–710, 2018.

R Tibshirani. Regression shrinkage and selection via the lasso. *Journal of the Royal Statistical Society B*, 58:267–288, 1996.

R Tibshirani. The lasso method for variable selection in the Cox model. *Statistics in Medicine*, 16:385–395, 1997.

MCK Tweedie. Functions of a statistical variate with given means, with special reference to Laplacian distributions. *Proceedings of the Cambridge Philosophical Society*, 13:41–49, 1947.

P Vallaisamy and D Sharma. Estimation of the mean of the selected gamma population. *Communications in Statistics–Theory and Methods*, 17: 2797–2817, 1988.

J van Gijn and A Algra. Ticlopidine, trials, and torture. *Stroke*, 25:1097–1098, 1994.

HC van Houwelingen. The role of empirical Bayes methodology as a leading principle in modern medical statistics. *Biometrical Journal*, 56:919–932, 2014.

TJ VanderWeele and MJ Knol. Interpretation of subgroup analyses in randomized trials: heterogeneity versus secondary interventions. *Annals of Internal Medicine*, 154:680–683, 2011.

R Varadhan and S J Wang. Standardization for subgroup analyses in clinical trials. *Journal of Biopharmaceutical Statistics*, 24:154–167, 2014.

R Varadhan and S J Wang. Treatment effect heterogeneity for univariate subgroups in clinical trials: Shrinkage, standardization, or else. *Biometrical Journal*, 58:133–153, 2016.

JH Venter. Estimation of the mean of the selected population. *Communication in Statistics–Theory and Methods*, 17:791–805, 1988.

S Wager, T Hastie, and B Efron. Confidence intervals for random forests: The jackknife and the infinitesimal jackknife. *Journal of Machine Learning Research*, 15:1625–1651, 2014.

H Wainer and H L Zwerling. Evidence that smaller schools do not improve student achievement. *Phi Delta Kappan*, 88:300–303, 2006.

A Wald. Tests of statistical hypotheses concerning several parameters when the number of observations is large. *Transactions of the American Mathematical Society*, 54:426–482, 1943.

J D Wallach, P G Sullivan, J F Trepanowski, K L Sainani, E W Steyerberg, and J P A Ioannidis. Evaluation of evidence of statistical support and corroboration of subgroup claims in randomized clinical trials. *JAMA Internal Medicine*, 177:554–560, 2017.

L Wallentin, R C Becker, A Budaj, C P Cannon, H Emanuelsson, H Katus, K W Mahaffey, B M Scirica, A Skene, P G Steg, R F Storey, and R A Harrington. Ticagrelor versus clopidogrel in patients with acute coronary syndromes. *New England Journal of Medicine*, 361:1045–1057, 2009.

L Wang, B Sherwood, and R Li. Comment. *Journal of the American Statistical Association*, 109:1007–1010, 2014.

R Wang, S W Lagakos, J H Ware, D J Hunter, and J M Drazen. Statistics in medicine—reporting of subgroup analyses in clinical trials. *New England Journal of Medicine*, 357:2189–2194, 2007.

H Wedel, D DeMets, P Deedwania, B Fagerberg, S Goldstein, S Gottlieb, A Hjalmarson, J Kjekshus, F Waagstein, and J Wikstrand. Challenges of subgroup analyses in multinational trials: Experiences from the MERIT-HF trial. *American Heart Journal*, 142:502–511, 2001.

X Su, CL Tsai, H Wang, D M Nickerson, and B Li. Subgroup analysis via recursive partitioning. *Journal of Machine Learning Research*, 10:141–158, 2009.

S Yusuf, R Collins, and R Peto. Why do we need some large, simple randomized trials? *Statistics in Medicine*, 3:409–422, 1984.

S Yusuf, J Wittes, J Probstfield, and HA Tyroler. Analysis and interpretation of treatment effects in subgroups of patients in randomized clinical trials. *Journal of the American Medical Association*, 266:93–98, 1991.

L Zhao, L Tian, T Cai, B Claggett, and LJ Wei. Effectively selecting a target population for a future comparative study. *Journal of the American Statistical Association*, 108:527–539, 2013.

Exploratory Subgroup Analyses in Clinical Research,
First Edition. Gerd Rosenkranz.
© 2020 John Wiley & Sons Ltd. Published 2020 by John Wiley & Sons Ltd.
Companion website: www.wiley.com/go/rosenkranz/exploratory

Index

Actimmune trial   10
aggregated estimator   132, 134, 142
Akaike information criterion (AIC)   70, 87, 138
apparent error   178, 180, 183, 186
average treatment effect   48, 148

backward elimination   110, 181
bagged estimator   145
bagging   131
Bayesian information criterion (BIC)   70, 87, 138, 140
best subset selection   86, 138

Beta-Blocker Heart Attack Trial (BHAT)   8, 64
bootstrap aggregating   131

causal inference   149
causal interaction   38
Clopidogrel versus aspirin in patients at risk of Ischemic events (CAPRI)   26, 53
confounding   17, 60, 84, 88
Consolidated Standards of Reporting Trials (CONSORT)   44
cross-validation   71, 88, 179

data dependent subset analysis   3

effect heterogeneity   38

empirical Bayes estimation 73, 92, 127
empirical Bayes estimator 95, 122
European Medicines Agency (EMA) 33, 42, 53
exchangeability 74, 93

false discovery rate 100, 123, 126
Food and Drug Administration (FDA) 4, 18, 19, 26, 27, 53
forward selection 86, 143, 159, 164, 181, 195

goodness-of-fit 70, 191
Gruppo Italiano per lo Studio della Streptochinasi nell'Infarcto (GISSI) 3

hierarchical model 32, 68, 73, 91
   estimation bias 104
   mixture prior 93, 111
   normal-normal 73, 124
   selection bias 106

ideal bootstrap 135
improper subgroup 34

infinitesimal jackknife estimator 136
Institute for Quality and Efficiency in Healthcare (IQWIQ) 26
interaction test 27, 33, 40
ISIS–2 5, 29, 64

law of small numbers 49
learning dataset 76, 131, 155, 176
Least absolute shrinkage and selection operator (Lasso) 87, 138, 152
   randomized 154, 161
link function 77, 83
log hazard ratio 74, 157
logit 77, 158
log odds ratio 74, 115, 157

mean squared error (MSE) 135, 154
metoprolol controlled release randomized intervention trial in heart failure (MERIT-HF) 20
Ministry of Health, Labor and Welfare (MHLW) 22
model error 178

modified outcome estimator 185
multiplicity 22, 33, 48
multivariate subgroup 37

National Institute of Health and Clinical Excellence (NICE) 26

personalized medicine 3
Pharmaceuticals and Medical Devices Agency (PMDA) 22
Platelet Inhibition and Clinical Outcomes Trial (PLATO) 20
post-hoc analyses 63
post-hoc subgroup 11, 18, 22, 59
potential outcome 79, 149
predefined subgroup 35
predicted individual treatment effect (PITE) 79, 148
  confidence interval 150
prediction 33, 69
  accuracy 70, 179
  prediction error 33, 69, 176, 181
predictive effect 36, 78
predictive subgroup 36

pre-specified subgroup 35, 43
probit 77
prognostic effect 36, 78
prognostic subgroup 36
proper subgroup 34
proportional hazards model 77, 86, 158

qualitative interaction 36, 79
quantitative interaction 20, 36

randomized lasso 154, 161
regression model 69, 85
regression to the mean 57
regularized estimator 87
Robbin's theorem 95, 127

Scheffé type confidence bounds 152
selection bias 33, 51, 107, 129
  and bootstrap 132
selective inference 153
Simpson's paradox 60
sparse model 85
subgroup
  multivariate 36
  predefined 35
  predictive 36
  prognostic 36

subgroup (*contd.*)
    univariate   36
statistical model   34, 85
Stein's theorem   72
stepwise selection   86

Therapeutic Arthritis Research and Gastrointestinal Event Trial (TARGET)   15

Trial Assigning Individualized Options for Treatment (TAYLORx)   17
Tweedie's formula   95

univariate subgroup   36

www.ingramcontent.com/pod-product-compliance
Lightning Source LLC
LaVergne TN
LVHW022003060526
838200LV00003B/76